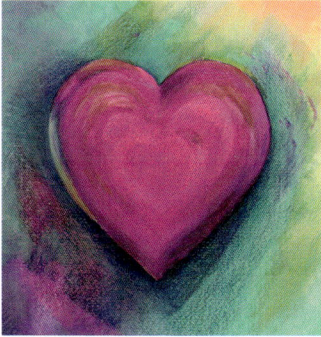

Healthy Living

2nd EDITION

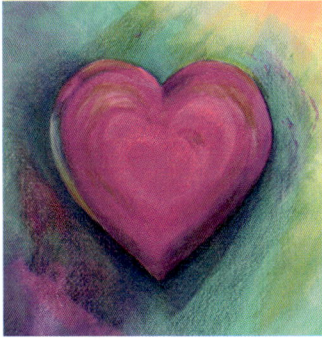

Healthy Living

2nd EDITION

VOLUME 3

SELF ESTEEM

MENTAL HEALTH

MENTAL ILLNESS

BEHAVIORS, HABITS, ADDICTIONS, AND EATING DISORDERS

Barbara Wexler

Elizabeth P. Manar, Project Editor

U·X·L
A part of Gale, Cengage Learning

GALE
CENGAGE Learning®

Detroit • New York • San Francisco • New Haven, Conn • Waterville, Maine • London

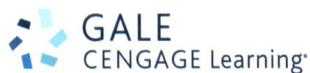

GALE CENGAGE Learning®

Healthy Living, 2nd Edition

Barbara Wexler

Project Editor: Elizabeth Manar

Managing Editor: Debra Kirby

Rights Acquisition and Management: Margaret Chamberlain-Gaston, Kimberly Potvin

Imaging and Multimedia: John L. Watkins

Composition: Evi Abou-El-Seoud, Mary Beth Trimper

Manufacturing: Wendy Blurton, Dorothy Maki

Product Managers: Douglas A. Dentino, Leigh Ann Cusack

Product Design: Kristine A. Julien

For product information and technology assistance, contact us at **Gale Customer Support, 1-800-877-4253**.
For permission to use material from this text or product, submit all requests online at **www.cengage.com/permissions**.
Further permissions questions can be emailed to **permissionrequest@cengage.com**

Cover photographs: Illustration of people and caduceus © Illustration Works/Corbis; illustration of person reaching for sun © Illustration Works/Corbis; illustration of vegetables in basket © Kain Zernitsky/Getty Images; and illustration of heart © Images.com/Corbis.

While every effort has been made to ensure the reliability of the information presented in this publication, Gale, a part of Cengage Learning, does not guarantee the accuracy of the data contained herein. Gale accepts no payment for listing; and inclusion in the publication of any organization, agency, institution, publication, service, or individual does not imply endorsement of the editors or publisher. Errors brought to the attention of the publisher and verified to the satisfaction of the publisher will be corrected in future editions.

LIBRARY OF CONGRESS CATALOGING-IN-PUBLICATION DATA

Wexler, Barbara.
  Healthy living / Barbara Wexler; Elizabeth P. Manar, project editor. — 2nd edition.
    v. cm
  Includes bibliographical references and index.
  Contents: volume 1. Personal hygiene — Nutrition — Physical fitness and exercise — Personal growth and development — Sexuality — volume 2. Environmental health — Preventative care and first aid — Medications — Mainstream medical system — Alternative medicine — volume 3. Self esteem — Mental health — Mental illness — Behaviors, habits, and addictions — Organizations.
  ISBN 978-1-4144-9865-2 (set : alk. paper) — ISBN 978-1-4144-9866-9 (v. 1 : alk. paper) — ISBN 978-1-4144-9867-6 (v. 2 : alk. paper) — ISBN 978-1-4144-9868-3 (v. 3 : alk. paper) — ISBN 978-1-4144-9869-0 (ebook)
  1. Health. 2. Health behavior. 3. Nutrition. I. Manar, Elizabeth P., editor. II. Title.
  RA776.W467 2013
  613—dc23   2012044096

Gale
27500 Drake Road
Farmington Hills, MI 48331-3535

978-1-4144-9865-2 (set)   1-4144-9865-9 (set)
978-1-4144-9866-9 (vol. 1)   1-4144-9866-7 (vol. 1)
978-1-4144-9867-6 (vol. 2)   1-4144-9867-5 (vol. 2)
978-1-4144-9868-3 (vol. 3)   1-4144-9868-3 (vol. 3)

This title is also available as an e-book.
ISBN-13: 978-1-4144-9869-0 (set)   ISBN-10: 1-4144-9869-1 (set)
Contact your Gale, a part of Cengage Learning, sales representative for ordering information.

Printed in the United States of America
1 2 3 4 5 6 7 17 16 15 14 13

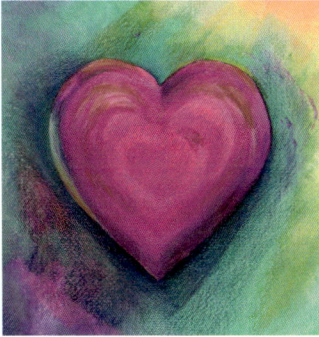

Contents

Reader's Guide vii

Words to Know xi

VOLUME 1

Nutrition 1

Physical Fitness and Exercise 43

Personal Care and Hygiene 77

Personal Growth and Development 113

Sexuality 143

VOLUME 2

Environmental Health 185

Preventive Care and First Aid 219

Medications 263

Mainstream Medical System 311

Alternative Medicine 367

VOLUME 3

Self Esteem 403

Mental Health 433

Mental Illness **483**

Behaviors, Habits, Addictions, and Eating Disorders **529**

List of Organizations .... **xxxvii**

Where to Learn More .... **xli**

General Index .... **li**

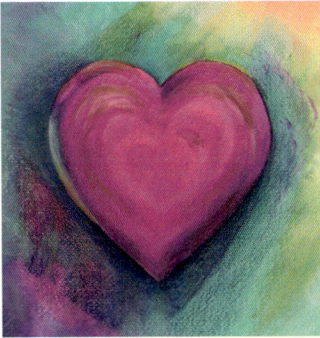

Reader's Guide

Healthy Living, 2nd Edition, covers a wide range of health-related topics and lifestyle issues in 14 chapters spread over three volumes. Each chapter is devoted to a specific health-related topic:

- Nutrition
- Physical Fitness and Exercise
- Personal Care and Hygiene
- Personal Growth and Development
- Sexuality
- Environmental Health
- Preventive Care and First Aid
- Medications
- Mainstream Medical System
- Alternative Medicine
- Self Esteem
- Mental Health
- Mental Illness
- Behaviors, Habits, Addictions, and Eating Disorders

Each chapter begins with a chapter-specific table of contents that outlines the main sections presented within the chapter. A brief overview then introduces readers to the topic at hand.

A "Words to Know" box included at the beginning of each chapter provides definitions of words and terms used in that chapter. At the end of each chapter, under the heading "For More Information," appears a list of books and Web sites that provide students with further information about that particular topic.

Health and safety tips, historical events, and other interesting facts relating to a particular topic are presented in sidebar boxes sprinkled throughout each chapter. More than 170 photos and illustrations enhance the text.

Each volume of *Healthy Living, 2nd Edition*, includes a comprehensive glossary collected from all the "Words to Know" boxes in the 14 chapters. A collective bibliography section and a list of organizations are included in each volume. A cumulative index providing access to all major terms and topics covered throughout *Healthy Living, 2nd Edition*, concludes each volume.

Comments and Suggestions

We welcome your comments on *Healthy Living, 2nd Edition*. Please write: Editors, *Healthy Living, 2nd Edition*, U•X•L, 27500 Drake Rd., Farmington Hills, Michigan, 48331-3535; call toll free: 1-800-877-4253; send fax to 248-699-8066; or send e-mail via http://www.gale.cengage.com

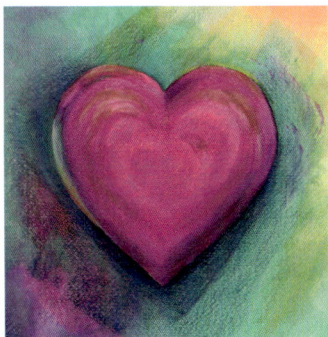

Please Read: Important Information

Healthy Living, 2nd Edition, is a medical reference product designed to inform and educate readers about health and lifestyle issues. U•X•L believes this product to be comprehensive, but not necessarily definitive. While U•X•L has made substantial efforts to provide information that is accurate and up to date, U•X•L makes no representations or warranties of any kind, including without limitation, warranties of merchantability or fitness for a particular purpose, nor does it guarantee the accuracy, comprehensiveness, or timeliness of the information contained in this product.

Readers should be aware that the universe of medical knowledge is constantly growing and changing, and that differences of medical opinion exist among authorities. They are also advised to seek professional diagnosis and treatment for any medical condition, and to discuss information obtained from this book with their health care provider.

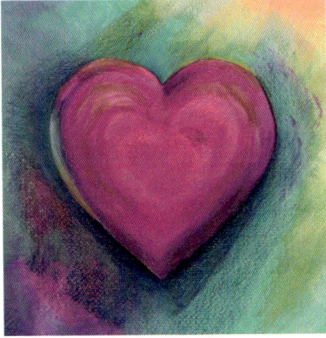

Words to Know

A

Abortion: The termination of a pregnancy by a surgical procedure or by prescription medication.

Abstinence: Restraining oneself from having sexual intercourse.

Abusive: Offensive, insulting, angry, or cruel.

Accredit: To recognize an educational institution for having the standards that allow graduates to practice in a certain field.

Acetaminophen: The generic name for a common nonprescription medication useful in the treatment of mild pain or fever.

Acid rain: Rain with a high content of sulfuric acid.

Acupuncture: A form of alternative medicine that involves stimulating certain points by putting very thin needles through the skin, to relieve pain, cure disease, and promote healing and overall well-being.

Adaptive behavior: The ways in which people adjust to new situations.

Addiction: The physical or mental need for a substance or the state of needing to compulsively repeat a behavior.

Adrenaline: Also known as epinephrine, adrenaline is a hormone that is released during times of stress that causes the heart rate to increase and strengthens the force of the heart's contraction. Secretion of adrenaline is part of the human "fight or flight" response to fear, panic, or perceived threat. Adrenaline also blocks the histamine response in an allergic reaction.

Adverse effect: The formal term for a harmful side effect of a drug or dietary supplement.

Advocate: A person who supports or defends a cause or a proposal.

Aerobic: Something that occurs in the presence of oxygen. Aerobic exercise strengthens the heart and lungs, improving the body's use of oxygen.

Affect: The expression of emotion or feelings displayed to others through facial expressions, hand gestures, voice tone, and other emotional signs.

Affectations: Artificial attitudes or behaviors.

Allopath: A doctor who advocates the conventional system of medical practice that uses measures that have proven to be effective to treat disease.

Allopathic: The system of medical practice making use of all measures that have proved to be effective in the treatment of disease.

Altered consciousness: A state of awareness that is different from typical, waking consciousness; often induced with the use of drugs and alcohol.

Alternative medicine: Medical practices that fall outside the spectrum of conventional allopathic medicine.

Alzheimer disease: A serious condition usually found in older adults that affects the parts of the brain that control thought, memory, and language.

Amenorrhea: The absence of menstrual cycles.

Amino acids: A group of 22 chemicals found in the human body that are the building blocks of proteins. Amino acids can be formulated in the laboratory and sold as dietary supplements in liquid, tablet, or powder form.

Anabolic steroids: Drugs that mimic the effects of male hormones in the body. They are used to build muscle tissue, increase appetite, and stimulate bone growth.

Anaerobic: Something that occurs without oxygen. Anaerobic exercise does not aim to improve the strength of the heart and lungs or the body's use of oxygen; instead it is exercise in which oxygen is used up more quickly than the body is able to replenish it. Weight training is an example of anaerobic exercise.

Analgesic: Any drug given to relieve pain.

Anemia: The condition of low iron in the blood.

Anhedonia: The inability to experience pleasure.

Anorexia nervosa: A term meaning "lack of appetite"; an eating disorder marked by a person's refusal or inability to maintain a healthy body weight resulting from restricting food intake or other means.

Antibiotic: A chemical substance that kills bacteria and stops their spread.

Antibiotics: A class of drugs that fight bacterial infections.

Antibodies: Proteins generally found in the blood that detect and destroy invaders, like bacteria, viruses, and fungi.

Antiemetics: Drugs that counteract or relieve nausea and vomiting.

Antihistamines: A class of drugs that counteract allergic responses.

Antioxidants: Powerful molecules found in certain foods and vitamins that help neutralize free radicals, which are damaging molecules.

Antipsychotic drugs: Drugs that reduce psychotic behavior, often having negative long-term side effects.

Antipyretic: A drug that works to lower fever.

Antitussive: A type of medication given to relieve coughing.

Anus: An opening in the body through which solid waste is expelled.

Anxiety: An abnormal and overwhelming sense of worry and fear that is often accompanied by physical reaction.

Appeal: To take a court's decision and have another higher court review it to either uphold or overturn the first decision.

Art therapy: The use of art and craft activities to treat emotional, mental, and physical disabilities.

Arthritis: Chronic inflammation and stiffness of the joints.

Artificial: Human-made; not found in nature.

Asbestos: A mineral fiber.

Associate's degree: Degree granted from two-year college institutions.

Attention-deficit / hyperactivity disorder (ADHD): A disorder that involves difficulty concentrating and overall inattentiveness.

B

Bachelor's degree: A four-year college degree.

Bacteria: Single-celled microorganisms, some of which are beneficial to the body while others cause disease.

Bedside manner: A physician's ability to put a patient at ease and communicate effectively.

Benign: Harmless; also, non-cancerous.

Binge-eating disorder: An eating disorder that involves repetitive episodes of binge eating in a restricted period of time over several months.

Bingeing: When an individual eats, in a particular period of time, an abnormally large amount of food.

Bioenergetics: Body/mind therapy that aims to free the body and the mind of negative actions.

Bioequivalence: The equality of two drug products in regard to dosage form, safety, strength, method of administration, quality, effectiveness, and intended use(s).

Biofeedback: The technique of teaching people to control involuntary bodily processes (such as heartbeats or brain waves).

Bladder: An organ that holds urine.

Blood pressure: The force of blood against the walls of blood vessels.

Blood vessel: Vessel through which blood flows.

Body set-point theory: The set point theory of weight control holds that the body will stay at a certain weight regardless of external factors, such as calorie intake or exercise.

Bonding: Attaching a material to the surface of a tooth for cosmetic purposes.

Botanical: Another term for a herbal or plant-based preparation or dietary supplement.

Bulimia nervosa: A term that means literally "ox hunger"; an eating disorder characterized by a repeated cycle of bingeing and purging.

Bullying: Unwanted, aggressive behavior that is repeated such as making threats, spreading rumors, attacking someone physically or verbally, and excluding someone from a group on purpose.

By-product: Something other than the main product that is produced in a chemical or biological process.

C

Caffeine: A bitter-tasting compound found in coffee and tea that acts as a stimulant.

Calcium: A mineral in the body that makes up much of the bones and teeth. Calcium helps nerve and muscle function, as well as the body's ability to convert food into energy.

Calorie: A unit of energy contained in the food and liquids that people consume.

Capitation: An agreement between a doctor and a managed care organization wherein the doctor is paid per person.

Carbohydrate: The body's primary energy source, carbohydrates are the body's fuel.

Carbon monoxide: A highly toxic, colorless, odorless gas that is produced whenever something is burned incompletely, or in a closed environment.

Carcinogenic: Cancer-causing.

Cardiovascular fitness: How efficiently the heart and lungs can pump blood (which holds oxygen) to muscles that are being worked.

Carve out: Medical services, such as substance abuse treatment, that are separated from the rest of the services within a health care plan.

Cervix: Narrow outer end of the uterus.

Chiropractic: Treating certain health conditions by manipulating and adjusting the spine.

Cholera: Any of several diseases of humans and domestic animals usually marked by severe gastrointestinal symptoms.

Cholesterol: A type of fat made in the body by the liver and also present in foods that come from animals, such as egg yolks, organ meats, and cheese.

Chromosome: Structures in cells that carry the genes that code for inherited characteristics.

Chronic condition: A condition that lasts a long time or occurs over and over again. Chronic conditions can be treated but not cured.

Chronic disease: An illness that is present for a long time or frequently recurs, such as diabetes or asthma.

Circumcision: The removal of the foreskin from the glans of the penis.

Classic conditioning: Learning involving an automatic response to a certain stimulus that is acquired and reinforced through association.

Clinical trial: An investigation of new drugs or treatment methods for specific diseases or conditions.

Clitoris: Small erectile organ at anterior part of the vulva.

Coexisting: Occurring at the same time.

Cognition: The mental processes of perception, recognition, conception, judgment, and reason.

Collagen: Fibrous protein found in connective tissues such as the skin and ligaments.

Compulsion: Habitual behaviors or mental acts an individual is driven to perform in order to reduce stress and anxiety brought on by obsessive thoughts.

Compulsive behavior: Behavior that is repeated over and over again, uncontrollably.

Conception: Also called fertilization. The formation of a cell capable of developing into a new being, such as when a man's sperm fertilizes a woman's egg to create a human embryo.

Confidence: Being certain and having a belief in one's own abilities.

Conflict: More than a disagreement, a conflict is a situation in which people feel that their well-being is threatened.

Congenital: Existing at birth.

Contaminate: To infect something or make something unsafe for use.

Continuing education: Formal schooling above and beyond any degree that is often required of medical professionals in order to keep practicing in their specific field.

Contraception: A birth control tool that prevents conception.

Copayment: A fixed amount of money that patients pay for each doctor's visit and for each prescription.

Correlation: The relation of two or more things that is not naturally expected.

Cosmic: Relating to the universe in contrast to Earth.

Cowper's glands: Two small glands on either side of the male urethra, below the prostate gland, that produce a clear, sticky fluid that is thought to coat the urethra for passage of sperm.

Crash: Coming down from being high on drugs or alcohol.

Credentials: Proof that a person is qualified to do a job.

Cruciform: The term for certain vegetables with long stems and branching tops, such as broccoli and cauliflower.

Cunnilingus: Oral stimulation of the vulva or clitoris.

Cut: The habit of mixing illegal drugs with another substance to produce a greater quantity of that substance.

Cuticle: The skin surrounding the nail.

Cyberbullying: Bullying that takes place using electronic technology such as e-mail, texts, and social networking sites.

D

Dance therapy: The use of dance and movement to treat or relieve symptoms associated with mental or physical illness.

Date rape: Also called acquaintance rape; forced sexual intercourse between a person and someone she or he is knows, is friends with, or is dating.

Deductible: The amount of money a patient must pay for services covered by the insurance company before the plan will pay for any medical bills.

Delirium: Mental disturbance marked by confusion, disordered speech, and even hallucinations.

Delusions: False or irrational beliefs people hold despite proof that their beliefs are untrue.

Dependent: A reliance on something or someone.

Depressed: Feeling sad, gloomy, and miserable.

Depression: A disorder marked by intense and prolonged feelings of sadness, emptiness, hopelessness, and irritability as well as a lack of pleasure in activities.

Detoxification: The process of freeing an individual of an intoxicating or addictive substance in the body or to free from dependence. Also, when doctors use medication to reduce or eliminate drugs or alcohol from a person's body.

Dextromethorphan (DXM): A cough suppressant drug found in many over-the-counter cough and cold medications. DXM is commonly abused as a recreational drug; in large doses it acts as a hallucinogen.

Diagnostic: Test used to recognize a disease or an illness.

Dietary supplement: As defined by the FDA, any vitamin, mineral, herb or plant (except tobacco), amino acid, or any extract or combination of these taken to complete a person's diet. The FDA regulates dietary supplements as food products rather than as medications.

Diuretic: A drug that increases the output of water from the body through urination.

DNA: Chromosomes are made of DNA, which is short for deoxyribonucleic acid.

Down syndrome: A form of mental retardation due to an extra chromosome present at birth, often accompanied by physical characteristics, such as sloped eyes.

Dream analysis: A technique of Freudian therapy that involves looking closely at dreams for symbolism and significance of themes and/or repressed thoughts.

Dysfunction: The inability to function properly.

Dyslexia: A disorder that centers on difficulties with word recognition.

E

Edema: Swelling.

Ego: The part of the personality that balances the drives of the id and the exterior world that is the center of the superego.

Ejaculation: Sudden discharge of fluid (from the penis).

Electrologist: A professional trained to perform electrolysis, the removal of hair using electric currents.

Electromagnetic: Magnetism developed by a current of electricity.

Electronic aggression: All types of violence that occur electronically.

Embryo: The two-month period after fertilization.

Emergency: The unexpected onset of a serious medical condition or life-threatening injury that requires immediate attention.

Emission: Substances released into the air.

Empathy: Understanding of another's situation and feelings.

Emphysema: A lung disease usually caused by smoking that produces shortness of breath and relentless coughing.

Enamel: The hard outer surface of the tooth.

Endocrine disrupter: Manmade chemical that can act like a naturally occurring hormone and disrupt normal hormonal cycles in animals and humans.

Endometrial: Referring to the lining of the uterus.

Endorphins: Any of a group of proteins in the brain and nervous system that act as the body's natural pain relievers. Some are released after exercise, causing people to feel better after exercise. Endorphins also affect emotions, helping people feel calm and content.

Endurance: A person's ability to continue doing a difficult activity without stopping for an extended period of time.

Enema: A process that expels waste from the body by injecting liquid into the anus.

Enuresis: The inability to control one's bladder while sleeping at night; bed-wetting.

Environment: The conditions and experiences that affect growth and development.

Environmental tobacco smoke (ETS): The mixture of the smoke from a lit cigarette, pipe, or cigar and the smoke exhaled by the person smoking; also known as secondhand smoke.

Enzyme: A complex protein found in the cells that acts as a catalyst for chemical reactions in the body.

Ephedra: An herb used in traditional Chinese medicine to treat asthma and hay fever, and used until recently in dietary supplements to improve athletic performance or produce short-term weight loss. The FDA banned the sale of ephedra in the United States in 2004 due to its potentially fatal side effects and its use in the production of methamphetamine.

Epidemic: The rapid spread of a disease to many people at the same time.

Epidemiology: The study of disease in a population.

Epididymis: System of ducts leading from the testes that holds sperm.

Esophagus: The muscular tube that connects the throat with the stomach.

Estrogen: Hormone that stimulates female secondary sex characteristics.

Euphoric: Having a feeling of well-being or elation.

Exercise: Physical activity that is structured, planned, and repetitive.

Exercise addiction: Also known as compulsive exercise, a condition in which participation in exercise activities is taken to an extreme; people exercise to the detriment of all other things in their lives.

Existential therapy: Therapy that stresses the importance of existence and urges patients to take responsibility for their psychological existence and well-being.

Expectorant: A type of medication given to help bring up mucus from the respiratory tract.

F

Fallopian tubes: Pair of tubes conducting the egg from the ovary to the uterus.

Fat: Part of every cell membrane and the most concentrated source of energy in one's diet, fat is used by the body to insulate, cushion, and support vital organs.

Fee-for-service: When a doctor or hospital is paid for each service performed.

Fellatio: Oral stimulation of the penis.

Fellowship: Advanced study and research that usually follows a medical residency.

Fertilization: Physically joining sperm and ovum.

Fetus: The developing baby from two months after fertilization until birth.

Fluoride: A chemical compound that is added to toothpaste and drinking water to help prevent tooth decay.

Formulary: A list of prescription drugs preferred by a health care plan for its members.

Free radicals: Harmful molecules in the body that damage normal cells and can cause cancer and other disorders.

Fungus: Any organism classified in the kingdom of Fungi (previously classified as members of the Plant kingdom, but lacking chlorophyll, flowers, or leaves). Mildew, mold, mushrooms, and yeasts are all types of fungus.

G

Gallstone: Stones made up of cholesterol or calcium that form in the gallbladder.

Gender: The roles, behaviors, activities, and attributes that a given society or culture considers appropriate for men and women.

Gene: Basic units of heredity that carry codes for individual traits.

Generativity: The ability or power to create, generate, or produce something.

Generic drug: A drug that is approved by the Food and Drug Administration but is marketed under its chemical name, rather than its brand name, and is less expensive than a brand name drug.

Genetic: Something present in the genes that is inherited from a person's biological parents.

Genetic disorder: A disease or condition caused by a problem with one or more genes.

Genetic predisposition: To be susceptible to a condition or disease because of genes.

Genetics: The scientific study of heredity that looks at how living things are similar and different from one another. Genetics helps to explain why children and many other living things look, sound, and often act like their parents.

Genitalia: The reproductive organs.

Genomics: The study of more than single genes, genomics looks at the functions of and the way all the genes in the genome work with one another.

Geriatric: Specializing in care of older adults.

Germs: A microorganism capable of causing disease.

Gestalt therapy: A humanistic therapy that urges individuals to satisfy growing needs, acknowledge previously unexpressed feelings, and reclaim facets of their personalities that have been denied.

Gingivitis: An inflammation of the gums that is the first stage of gum disease.

Gland: A part of the body that makes a fluid that is either used or excreted by the body; glands make sweat and bile.

H

Habit: A behavior or routine that is repeated.

Halitosis: Chronic bad breath caused by poor oral hygiene, illness, or another condition.

Hallucinations: The perception of seeing or hearing things when they aren't really present.

Hallucinogens: A group of drugs and plant-derived substances that induce changes in thinking, perception, and consciousness as well as mood.

Hangnail: Loose skin near the base of the nail.

Hangover: The syndrome that occurs after being high on drugs or drinking alcohol, often including nausea, headache, dizziness, and fuzzy-mindedness.

Heart disease: Problems with the heart or blood vessels, such as thickening of the arteries or a build-up of cholesterol and fat in artery walls, which can lead to heart attack.

Heat stroke: A serious condition that causes the body to stop sweating and become dangerously overheated.

Hemoglobin: A protein found in red blood cells, needed to carry oxygen to the body's many tissues.

Hemorrhoids: Enlarged and swollen veins in the anus that may bleed.

Hepatitis: One of several severe liver-damaging diseases specified by the letters A, B, C and D.

Herbicide: A chemical agent used to kill plants, such as weeds.

Heredity: The passing of characteristics from parents to their children.

Histamines: Chemicals released in an allergic reaction that cause swelling of body tissues. Histamines are responsible for some allergy symptoms like runny nose, itching, and sneezing.

Holistic: Of or relating to the whole rather than a specific part or disorder; holistic medicine treats both the mind and the body.

Homeopathy: A system of natural remedies that relies on the idea that "like cures like."

Hormones: Chemicals produced by the body's glands that regulate various bodily functions, such as growth.

Human genome: All the genetic information in a person.

Humane: Marked by compassion or sympathy for other people or creatures.

Humanistic: A philosophy that places importance on human interests and dignity, stressing the individual over the religious or spiritual.

Hymen: Fold of mucous membrane partly closing the orifice of the vagina.

Hypertension: High blood pressure.

Hypnosis: A trance-like state of consciousness brought about by suggestions of relaxation, which is marked by increased suggestibility.

Hypoallergenic: Unlikely to cause an allergic reaction.

Hypothesize: To make a tentative assumption in order to test its logical or observable consequences.

I

Id: According to Sigmund Freud, the biological instincts that revolve around pleasure, especially sexual and aggressive impulses.

Immune system: The body's system of natural defenses that helps the body resist harmful substances or microorganisms—bacteria, viruses, parasites, and fungi.

Immunization: The introduction of disease-causing compounds into the body in very small amounts in order to allow the body to form antigens against the disease.

Incinerator: A machine that burns waste materials.

Indemnity plan: A plan in which the insurance company sets a standard amount that it will pay for specific medical services.

Industrial: Relating to a company that manufactures a product.

Inert: A chemical agent lacking in active properties.

Infection: A disease caused by an invasion of bacteria, viruses, or fungi.

Infinitesimals: Immeasurably small quantity or variable.

Inhalants: Substances that people sniff to get high.

Inherent: Belonging to the essential nature of something.

Insight therapy: Therapy techniques that assume that a patient's behavior, thoughts, and emotions become disordered as the result of a lack of understanding of what motivates them.

Insomnia: Chronic sleeplessness or sleep disturbances.

Insulin: The substance in the body that regulates blood sugar levels.

Intelligence quotient (IQ): A standardized measure of a person's mental ability as compared to those in his or her age group.

Internalized: To incorporate something into one's self.

Internship: Supervised practical experience.

Intestinal: Having to do with the intestine, the part of the body that digests food.

Iridology: The study of the iris of the eye in order to diagnose illness or disease.

Iron-deficiency anemia: When the body is lacking in the right amount of red blood cells, caused by a deficiency of iron.

Irrational: Lacking reason or understanding.

J

Judgmental: A tendency to pass judgment and sometimes to judge harshly.

K

Keratin: A tough protein produced by the body that forms the hair and nails.

Kidney stone: Stones made of calcium or other minerals that form in the kidney or the ureter, a tube that leads to the bladder.

Kinesiology: The study of anatomy in relation to movement of the body.

Kleptomania: Habitual stealing.

L

Labia majora: Outer fatty folds of the vulva (big lips).

Labia minora: Inner connective folds of the vulva (little lips).

Lanugo: Fine hair that grows all over the body to keep it warm when the body lacks enough fat to accomplish this.

Larynx: The upper part of the trachea that contains the vocal cords that make speech possible. Also called the voice box.

Laxatives: Medications that are given to treat constipation by inducing bowel movements. They may work by increasing the bulk of the stool, holding water within the stool, softening the stool, or stimulating the intestines to contract more vigorously.

Leaching: The process of dissolving outward by the action of a permeable substance.

Lead: A heavy, flexible metallic element that is often used in pipes and batteries.

Learning disorders: Developmental problems relating to speech, academic, or language skills that are not linked to a physical disorder or mental retardation.

Licensed: Authorization to practice a certain occupation.

M

Mantra: A phrase repeated during meditation to center the mind.

Manual: Involving the hands.

Massage therapy: The manipulation of soft tissue in the body with the aim of relieving and preventing pain, stress, and muscle spasms.

Master's degree: A college degree that ranks above a four-year bachelor's degree.

Masturbation: Erotic stimulation of one's own genital organs.

Maturation: Process of becoming mature; developing, growing up.

Medicaid: The joint state-federal health care program for low-income people.

Medicare: The federal health insurance program for older adults and people with disabilities.

Medigap: Private insurance that helps pay for some of the costs of care that are not covered by Medicare.

Meditation: A practice that helps one to center and focus the mind; sometimes used to help recovering addicts.

Menstruation: Monthly shedding of the lining of the uterus in females, which results in the discharge of blood and tissue.

Metabolism: The rate at which the body uses energy.

Microscopic: Invisible without the use of a microscope, an instrument that enlarges images of tiny objects.

Mineral: A nutrient that helps regulate cell function and provides structure for cells.

Modeling: Learning based on modeling one's behavior on that of another person.

Monosodium glutamate (MSG): A substance that enhances flavor but causes food intolerance in some people.

Mortality: The number of deaths in a given time or place.

Mucous membranes: The lining of the nose and sinus passages that helps shield the body from allergens and germs.

Musculoskeletal: Relating to the muscles and bones.

Music therapy: The use of music to treat or relieve symptoms of certain mental or physical illnesses.

Mutation: A change in the genetic material.

N

Narcotic: Originally, any drug that induces sleep; in modern usage, any drug derived from opium whose use is prohibited by law or has a high potential for abuse and dependence.

National health care system: A system in which the government provides medical care to all its citizens.

Naturopathy: A kind of alternative medicine that focuses on the body's inherent healing powers and works with those powers to restore and maintain overall health.

Neurosis: An emotional disorder that produces fear and anxiety.

Nitrogen dioxide: A gas that cannot be seen or smelled. It irritates the eyes, ears, nose, and throat.

Noninvasive: Not involving penetration of the skin.

Nonsteroidal anti-inflammatory drugs (NSAIDs): Anti-inflammatory drugs that work by inhibiting the production of prostaglandins (a group of compounds that affect various bodily processes). Aspirin is the most familiar NSAID.

Nutrient: A food substance that nourishes the body.

O

Obesity: The condition of being very overweight, marked by too much body fat.

Obsessions: Repeating thoughts, impulses, or mental images that are irrational and uncontrollable.

Off-label use: The practice of prescribing a medication for use unapproved (or not yet approved) by the FDA.

Operant conditioning: Learning that involves a voluntary response to a certain stimuli based on positive or negative consequences resulting from the response.

Opioids: A group of powerful pain relievers either derived directly from the opium poppy or from semi-synthetic compounds related to opium. They have a high potential for abuse.

Oral sex: Sexual activity involving the mouth.

Osteopathy: A system of medical practice based on the theory that disease is due chiefly to mechanical misalignment of bones or body parts.

Osteoporosis: A degenerative bone disease that causes a decrease in bone mass, making bones more brittle and fragile and likely to break.

Ova: Female reproductive cells; also called eggs.

Ovaries: Female reproductive organs that produce eggs and female sex hormones.

Overdose: A dangerous, often deadly, reaction to taking too much of a certain drug.

Ovulation: Discharge of mature ovum from the ovary.

Ovum: The female reproductive cell.

Oxycodone: A semi-synthetic opioid drug prescribed for the relief of moderate to severe pain. Sold under the trade name OxyContin, it is one of the most commonly abused prescription drugs in the United States and Canada.

Ozone layer: The atmospheric shield that protects the planet from harmful ultraviolet radiation.

P

Parasite: An organism that lives on or inside another organism at the expense of its host.

Parkinson disease: A progressive disease that causes slowing and stiffening of muscular activity, trembling hands, and a difficulty in speaking and walking.

Particle: A miniscule pollutant released when fuel does not burn completely.

Peers: People who are the same age, status, or ability or those in the same social group.

Penis: Male sex organ and channel by which urine and ejaculate leave the body.

Perception: One's consciousness and way of observing things.

Periodontal disease: Gum disease, the first stage of which is gingivitis.

Pesticide: A chemical agent used to kill bugs.

Pharmacotherapy: The use of medication to treat emotional and mental problems.

Phobia: A form of an anxiety disorder that involves intense and illogical fear of an object or situation.

Physical activity: Any movement that spends energy.

Physiological: Relating to the functions and activities of life on a biological level.

Physiology: A branch of science that focuses on the functions of the body.

Pinna: Outer part of the ear; part of the ear that is visible.

Placenta: Tissue lining the uterus that provides food and oxygen to the developing fetus and embryo.

Plaque: A sticky film of bacteria that grows around the teeth.

Plaster: A medicated or protective dressing that consists of a film (as of cloth or plastic) usually spread with a medicated substance.

Point of service: A health plan in which members can see the doctor of their choosing at the time they need to see a doctor.

Pores: Small openings in the skin.

Post-traumatic stress disorder (PTSD): Reliving trauma and anxiety related to an event that occurred earlier.

Potassium: A chemical element that is a silver-white, soft metal occurring in nature.

Predisposition: To be susceptible to something.

Preferred provider organization: A health plan in which members have their health care paid for only when they choose from a network of specific doctors and hospitals.

Premium: Consideration paid for a contract of insurance.

Prescription: A physician or other health care professional's written directions for the preparation, dispensing, and use of a medication or medical device.

Preventive care: Medical care, such as immunizations, that helps to prevent disease.

Primary care physician: The doctor who is responsible for the total care of a patient and refers patients to other doctors or specialists.

Pro-choice: Supports a woman's choice in regard to abortion.

Prostate gland: A muscular glandular body situated at the base of the male urethra.

Protein: An organic substance made of amino acids that are necessary for human life.

Protozoan: One-celled organism that can cause disease in humans.

Pseudoephedrine: A compound commonly found in cold or allergy medications to relieve nasal or sinus congestion. Its purchase is restricted in the United States because it can be used to make methamphetamine.

Psychiatry: The branch of medicine that relates to the study and treatment of mental illness.

Psychoactive: Something that affects brain function, mood, and behavior.

Psychoanalysis: A theory of psychotherapy, based on the work of Sigmund Freud, involving dream analysis, free association, and different facets of the self (id, ego, superego).

Psychodrama: A therapy that involves a patient enacting or reenacting life situations in order to gain insight and change behavior. The patient is the actor while the therapist is the director.

Psychodynamics: The forces (emotional and mental) that develop in early childhood and how they affect behavior and mental well-being.

Psychological vulnerability: Used to describe people who may be at risk for drug addiction because of prior experiences or other influences.

Psychology: The scientific study of mental processes and behaviors.

Psychotherapy: Treatment during which a trained mental health professional tries to help a patient resolve emotional and mental distress.

Puberty: The onset of sexual maturation, during which adolescents develop characteristics of their sex and become capable of reproduction.

Purging: When a person gets rid of the food that she has eaten by vomiting, taking an excessive amount of laxatives, diuretics, or enemas or engaging in fasting and/or excessive exercise.

Pyromania: Habitual need to start fires.

Q

Qi (or chi): Life energy vital to an individual's well-being.

R

Radiation: Energy or rays emitted when certain changes occur in the atoms or molecules of an object or substance.

Radon: A colorless, odorless, radioactive gas produced by the naturally occurring breakdown of the chemical element uranium in soil or rocks.

Rational-emotive behavior therapy: Therapy that seeks to identify a patient's irrational beliefs as the key to changing behavior rather than examining the cause of the conflict itself.

Rationing: The process of limiting certain products or services because of a shortage.

Reality therapy: A therapy that empowers people to make choices and control their destinies.

Referral: A request from the primary care physician for a patient to see another doctor, usually a specialist in a specific area of medicine.

Reflexology: A type of bodywork that involves applying pressure to certain points, referred to as reflex points, on the foot.

Registered: To complete the standards of education issued by a state government to practice a certain profession.

Reimbursement plan: A plan in which a patient must pay for medical services up front and then is paid back by the insurance company.

Remorse: Sadness and regret stemming from guilt over past actions.

Residency: Advanced training in a medical specialty that includes or follows a physician's internship.

Residential treatment: Treatment that takes place in a facility in which patients reside.

Reye's syndrome: A disorder primarily found in children that principally affects the liver and brain, and is marked by the rapid development of life-threatening neurological symptoms. It is thought to be associated with giving aspirin during the course of a fever-producing illness, but the exact connection is not known as of 2012.

Right-to-life: Supports anti-abortion (with possible exceptions for incest and rape) movement.

Ritual: Observances or ceremonies that mark change, renewal, or other events.

Russell's sign: Calluses, cuts, and sores on the knuckles from repeated self-induced vomiting.

S

Saturated fat: Fat that is solid at room temperature.

Savant: A person with extensive knowledge in a very specific area.

Schizophrenia: A chronic psychological disorder marked by scattered, disorganized thoughts, confusion, and delusions.

Scrotum: External pouch that contains the testes.

Sebum: An oily substance that lubricates the hair shaft.

Sectarian medicine: Medical practices not based on scientific experience; also known as alternative medicine.

Sedative: Any drug given to help a person sleep or to calm or relax a patient before surgery.

Self-concept: The view that a person holds of him- or herself.

Self-esteem: How a person feels about him- or herself.

Self-medicate: When a person treats an ailment, mental or physical, with alcohol or drugs rather than seeing a physician or mental health professional.

Self talk: The ongoing internal conversations people have with themselves, which influence how they feel and behave.

Sexual abuse: All levels of sexual contact against anyone's will, including inappropriate touching, kissing, and intercourse.

Sexual harassment: All unwanted and unsolicited sexual advances, talk, and behavior.

Sexual intercourse: Involves genital contact between individuals.

Sibling: Brothers and sisters who have at least one parent in common.

Smegma: Cheesy sebaceous matter that collects between the penis and the foreskin.

Social norms: Standard practices that are largely accepted by society.

Social Security: A federal government program that provides benefits to retired persons, the unemployed, and the disabled.

Somatogenesis: Originating in the body, as opposed to the mind.

Specialist: A doctor who concentrates on only one area of medicine, such as a dermatologist (skin specialist).

Species: A group whose members can breed to produce offspring.

Sperm: The male reproductive cell.

Stagnation: A state of inactivity; failing to grow, change, or develop.

Sterilization: A process that makes something free of living bacteria.

Stimulant: A type of drug given to increase alertness or wakefulness, or to improve concentration.

Stressor: Something (for example, an event) that causes physical or emotional stress.

Subatomic: Relating to particles smaller than atoms.

Suicide: Taking one's own life.

Sulfur dioxide: A toxic gas that can also be converted to a colorless liquid.

Superego: According to Sigmund Freud, the part of one's personality that is concerned with social values and rules.

Suppository: A conical or bullet-shaped solid medication inserted into the rectum or vagina, designed to melt at body temperature and release its active ingredient into the body through the mucous membranes.

Suppress: To stop the development or growth of something.

Symptom: Something that indicates the presence of an illness or bodily disorder.

Synthetic: Something that is human-made; not found in nature.

T

Tamper-evident packaging (TEP): Protective packaging devices mandated by the FDA for over-the counter-medications since 1983. TEP alerts customers that an OTC may have been intentionally altered or contaminated in some way. TEP includes outer shrink wrapping over the caps and necks of bottles; plastic seals over the ends of cardboard boxes; inner foil seals over the opening of tablet containers; blister packaging of tablets and capsules; and similar devices.

Tartar: When plaque on the teeth hardens due to mineral deposits and makes it harder to remove from the teeth.

Tendinitis: Inflammation of the tissue that connects muscles to bones.

Testicles: Male reproductive gland that produces sperm.

Testosterone: Hormone produced by testes.

Thyroid: A gland that controls the growth of the body.

Tic: A quirk of behavior or speech that happens frequently and repeatedly.

Tolerance: The build-up of resistance to the effects of a substance.

Topical: Referring to a medication applied directly to the surface of the body (skin, hair, scalp, or nails).

Tourette's Disorder: A disorder marked by the presence of multiple motor tics and at least one vocal tic, as well as compulsions and hyperactivity.

Toxic: Relating to or caused by a poison.

Toxin: A poison made by a germ.

Transdermal: Referring to a medication that is delivered to the body by being absorbed through the skin.

U

Ultrasound: The use of high-frequency sound waves to form an image to detect a problem in the body.

Umbilical cord: The tube that connects the fetus to its mother and delivers food and oxygen from the placenta to the fetus.

Unsaturated fat: Fat that is liquid at room temperature, like vegetable oil.

Uranium: A chemical element that is a silver-white, hard metal and is radioactive.

Urethra: The tube from the bladder to the outside of the body through which urine is expelled.

Uterus: Womb; female organ that contains and nourishes an embryo/fetus.

V

Vaccine: A substance made up of weak or killed bacteria or viruses given to help prevent infectious diseases.

Vagina: The female canal that leads from the cervix (or opening of the uterus) to the vulva (or the external female genitalia).

Vas deferens: Spermatic duct connected to the epididymis and seminal vesicle.

Vegan: A strict vegetarian who doesn't eat any animal by-products or any dairy products or eggs.

Vegetarian: A person who lives on a diet free of meat products; some vegetarians will eat eggs or dairy products, while others will not.

Veneer: A covering, often made of porcelain, that is placed over a tooth that is damaged or for cosmetic reasons.

Vertebra: A bony piece of the spinal column fitting together with other vertebrae to allow flexible movement of the body. (The spinal cord runs through the middle of each vertebra.)

Virus: A tiny organism that causes disease.

Vitamin: A nutrient that enables the body to use fat, protein, and carbo-hydrates effectively.

Volatile organic compound (VOC): An airborne chemical that contains carbon.

Vulva: External parts of the female genital organs.

W

Withdrawal: The phase of removal of drugs or alcohol from the system of the user.

Y

Yang: In Chinese traditional medicine, one of the opposite forces (along with yin) that make up all things, including the human body.

Yin: In Chinese traditional medicine, one of the opposite forces (along with yang) that make up all things, including the human body.

Yoga: A form of exercise and a system of health that incorporates a series of exercises utilizing regulated breathing, concentration, physical postures, and flexibility.

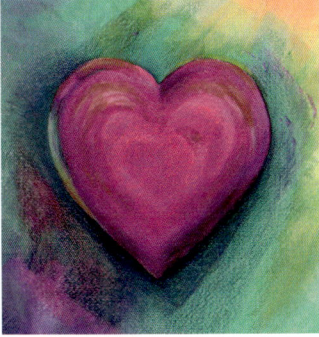

Self-Esteem

Introduction **405**

Developing Self-Concept **406**

Low Self-Esteem **412**

Healthy Self-Esteem **415**

Friends Can Help or Harm Self-Esteem **417**

Avoid Actions and Behaviors That Harm Self-Esteem **420**

Violent Behavior **421**

Building Self-Esteem **425**

For More Information **430**

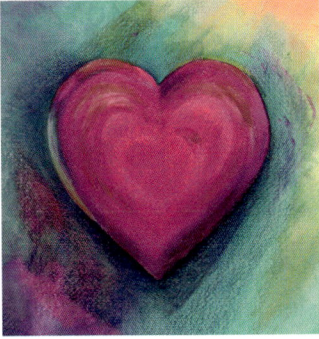

Self-Esteem

Self-esteem is the way a person feels about him- or herself. Self-esteem is a person's feeling and judgment about his or her own worth and value. It takes into account how a person feels about his or her appearance, accomplishments, abilities, beliefs, emotions, and behaviors. Self-esteem is related to self-respect and self-confidence. Self-esteem is considered a personality trait, which means that it while it can change somewhat, it generally does not change dramatically or very much throughout life.

Self-concept is related to self-esteem but it is not the same as self-esteem. It's not how a person feels about him- or herself, it is the actual way that people see themselves—how they would describe themselves and how they believe others view them. For teens, self-concept arises from feelings about how they are doing in school, socially—how they get along with friends—athletically, and in other aspects of life. Self-esteem is a teen's overall evaluation of him- or herself, including feelings of general happiness and satisfaction.

For example, a teenager might describe herself as honest, happy, athletic, and creative, or smart, funny, organized, and optimistic. Self-concept may be realistic, which means the person's description of him- or herself is accurate and pretty close to how others would describe the person, or it may be unrealistic, which means that it doesn't accurately describe the persons' strengths and weaknesses.

Teens often have unrealistic self-concepts. They may not appreciate their strengths and may be very self-critical about qualities they believe are faults or weaknesses. It is common for teens to focus on weaknesses rather than strengths and even to exaggerate the faults they find in themselves. For example, a teen that is shorter than others his age may focus on his height and how it prevents him from doing as well as he would like in sports. Teen girls and boys often exaggerate the importance of a physical feature they are unhappy about, such as glasses, big ears, or curly hair, so that it overshadows all of their other strengths.

Words to Know

Abusive: Offensive, insulting, angry, or cruel.

Adrenaline: Also known as epinephrine, adrenaline is a hormone that is released during times of stress that causes the heart rate to increase and strengthens the force of the heart's contraction. Secretion of adrenaline is part of the human "fight or flight" response to fear, panic, or perceived threat. Adrenaline also blocks the histamine response in an allergic reaction.

Bullying: Unwanted, aggressive behavior that is repeated such as making threats, spreading rumors, attacking someone physically or verbally, and excluding someone from a group on purpose.

Confidence: Being certain and having a belief in one's own abilities.

Conflict: More than a disagreement, a conflict is a situation in which people feel that their well being is threatened.

Cyberbullying: Bullying that takes place using electronic technology such as e-mail, texts, and social networking sites.

Depressed: Feeling sad, gloomy, and miserable.

Electronic aggression: All types of violence that occur electronically.

Judgmental: A tendency to pass judgment and sometimes to judge harshly.

Peers: People who are the same age, status, or ability or those in the same social group.

Self-concept: The view that a person holds of him- or herself.

Self-esteem: How a person feels about him- or herself.

Self talk: The ongoing internal conversations people have with themselves, which influence how they feel and behave.

Sibling: Brothers and sisters who have at least one parent in common.

This chapter describes how self-concept develops, ways to build and support self-esteem, threats to self-esteem, and the relationship between self-esteem and health. It defines and describes high self-esteem, low self-esteem, and healthy self-esteem. It also suggests ways that people can help one another to feel happier and more satisfied with themselves and more confident in their abilities.

Developing Self-Concept

Self-concept develops early in life as a result of relationships with other people. People develop their opinions about themselves by seeing how others respond to and communicate with them. These other people act like mirrors, and the images they reflect help to form self-concept.

Family relationships with parents, sisters, brothers, and even extended family and other caregivers are the first influences on self-concept. Self-concept and self-esteem are formed soon after birth as infants learn that parents or caregivers will meet their needs for nourishment, love, comfort, closeness, and attention. When their needs are met, infants feel secure; this feeling of security is the foundation for self-concept and self-esteem.

When parents express love and support for their children, the children generally develop positive self-concepts. On the other hand, children with parents or caregivers who often neglect or criticize them, speak harshly to them, or are abusive are more likely to develop negative self-concepts.

A young child's self concept is usually very simple and descriptive. It's usually just the facts—the child's name, age, gender, and physical attributes. "I am Kate and I am 4. I have brown hair, brown eyes, and a baby brother." The young child doesn't usually make judgments about the qualities described.

Young children develop their self-concepts by mastering a variety of skills and tasks. Each accomplishment, such as learning to solve problems, dressing on their own, or riding a tricycle gives them a sense of mastery. This sense of mastery, along with their parents' and siblings' responses to them, helps to shape their self concepts.

Over time, other people influence the development of self-concept. The ability to make friends with peers (children of the same age) influences how children view themselves and understand their place in the world outside of their families. Friends, teachers, athletic coaches, and others who support and encourage or ignore and discourage children and teens all help to shape self-concept.

As children get older and become teens, they better understand how others view their skills and are better at telling the difference between their efforts and abilities. As a result, their self-perceptions and self-concepts become more accurate.

These important relationships, with parents, teachers, and friends, help people develop an understanding of themselves, and they begin to be judgmental, deciding which characteristics and qualities are good and which are bad. A teenager may decide, "I am good at math and science," and "I am having trouble learning to draw—I don't think I'll be an artist," or "The coach has me pitching more often—I must be getting better," and "I think the girl who sits behind me in English class likes me."

Healthy Living, 2nd Edition

As people age, the opinions of others continue to influence self-concept, but not as much as they do during childhood and the teen years. Older children and teens often find out that parents are concerned with how well they do in school and their behavior at home and at school, while their friends often value physical appearance and athletic skill more than academics.

Support from parents and friends and other peers is particularly important to teenagers' self-concept. When children are young, approval from parents is more important in shaping self-concept than approval from peers. The influence of friends and peers increases over the course of development, but the influence of parents does not decrease. Teens' views of the support they receive from parents and peers are even more important to self-concept than the actual strength or amount of support given them.

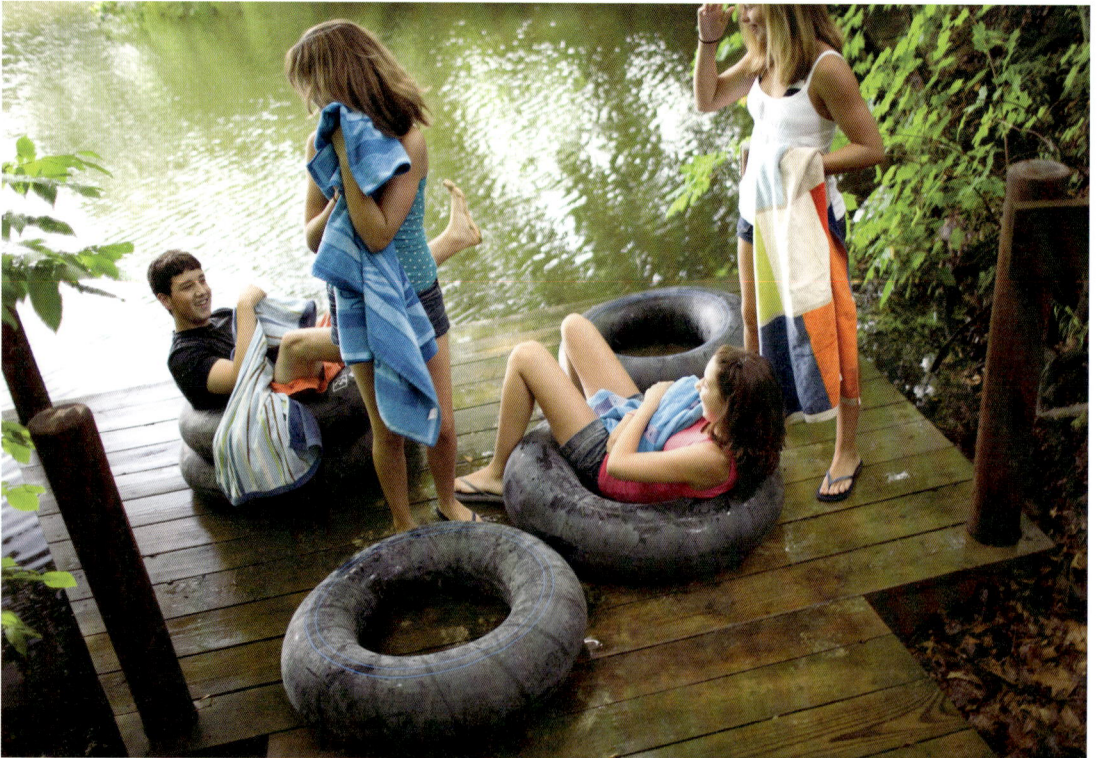

As children move into the teen years, the opinions of their peers become more important and may become a positive or negative influence on self-esteem. © PVSTOCK.COM/ALAMY.

Throughout their lives, adults continue to use the opinions of others to help them to understand themselves. Although their parents' opinions are still important, adults' self concepts are more likely to be influenced by their husbands, wives, or partners, coworkers and bosses, and friends.

There also are other influences on self-concept, like the media. Images in magazines, on television, in movies, and on the Internet tell people what they should look like and what they should be doing, which in turn shapes people's feelings about themselves. For example, many girls and young women compare themselves to photos of models and celebrities that have been airbrushed and retouched. By comparing themselves to these unreal and unrealistic images, it is easy to understand why they might feel badly about themselves and how they look.

Although teens—girls and boys—tend to base their views about attractiveness on celebrities and media figures, it is important for them to understand that it is unrealistic and unhealthy to compare themselves to celebrities or the images they see in the media.

Families Help Shape Self-Concept Humans are social beings and as such, have a need to belong. A family is the first group people belong to. Families are important social groups. They usually consist of two or more people who share a home as well as common goals and values. Families pass on and teach their values to children. Children learn their first social skills in their families, and their families help them to form their self-concept. They develop a sense of who they are and their place in the family.

Today, families come in many different shapes and sizes. But members of families have special relationships. Generally, the adults in the family provide food, clothing, shelter, and emotional support for the children. Adults also teach children and help them learn about themselves and the world around them.

There are many different kinds of families. A nuclear family, traditionally considered the basic unit of society, is a mother and father and their children. But a couple without any children is also a family. And an unmarried couple with children is also a family. Today, many families have only one parent. The number of single-parent families has grown in recent years. Nearly one-third of families in the United States are headed by one parent. The parent may be single, divorced, or widowed.

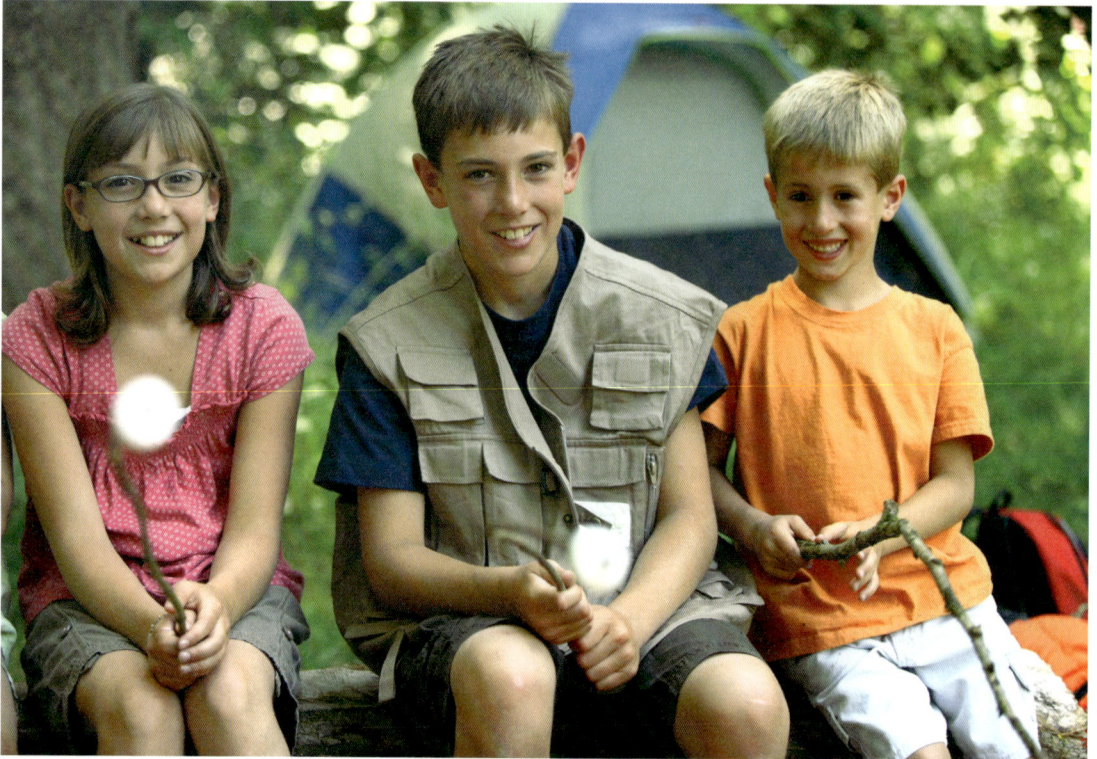

Siblings are some of the first people to give one a sense of self-concept. Having a supportive, loving family environment helps shape positive self-concept. © MORGAN LANE PHOTOGRAPHY/SHUTTERSTOCK.COM.

There also are cross-generational families such as families headed by grandparents who are raising their grandchildren. Extended families are nuclear families or single parent families and other relatives. Extended families may include grandparents, aunts, uncles, nieces, nephews, and step-children. Blended families are made up of a parent, stepparent, and children of one or both parents.

Other families include adopted and foster children. Still others have same-sex parents. In the United States, about eight million children live in families with same sex parents.

Family Problems At one point or another, practically all families have to cope with challenges and problems. Sometimes families facing problems can handle the problems by themselves, and other times they may need help. School counselors, teachers, members of the clergy, doctors, nurses, social service agencies, and family counselors can help to support families facing serious problems. Youth leaders, who lead groups of scouts, 4-H clubs, and YMCA/YWCA groups, also can help teens and families with problems.

Some of the most common problems families face include illness and disability, unemployment, separation and divorce, and moving.

When a family member is ill or injured, the family often must spend time caring for the person who is ill. This can disrupt normal family life, and children and teens may have to pitch in and help more than they usually do with household chores. When a child is sick or has a disability, at times other children in the family may feel neglected because their parents are focusing on caring for the child who is ill or has a disability.

When a family member is suffering from an illness such as substance abuse or a serious mental health problem, it may be even more stressful than when caring for someone who is sick or injured. People with mental health or substance abuse problems like alcoholism or drug addiction may behave differently from day to day. Not knowing how a parent or sibling is going to act or behave can be very scary.

In recent years, many families have suffered from job loss, unemployment, and trouble paying bills. This is very stressful for everyone in the family and sometimes means the family must move or change how they live. Even when moving is not the result of job loss, it can be difficult for the family. Adjusting to a new state, city, or even just a new neighborhood takes awhile. Going to a new school and having to make new friends can be scary and challenging.

Another common family challenge is military deployment. When a parent or adult child must be away for months at a time, family life may be disrupted. The remaining parent and older children and teens may have to take on additional responsibilities and the family may be anxious when waiting to hear from the person who is serving in the military. Military families also worry about the safety and well being of their loved one.

Separation and divorce are problems many families face. When parents decide to separate it is very stressful for the entire family. Children may feel their lives are being turned upside down as they adjust to new living arrangements. When divorcing parents argue about which parent children will live with, how often the children will visit with the other parent, and other arrangements, children may feel confused, angry, and frightened.

Healthy Living, 2nd Edition

Another serious problem that can affect families is abuse. Abuse can be physical like hitting, punching, kicking, or slapping, or it may be emotional—mean and cruel behavior, threats and yelling, as well as constant teasing and being overly critical. A family member may neglect or mistreat one or more family members. Neglect may be not providing children with the food and clothing they need or it may be emotional neglect—failing to provide the emotional support and caring that family members need to feel safe, cared for, and secure.

Low Self-Esteem

Self-concept is closely linked to self-esteem. Self-esteem is the personal pride and confidence that people feel in their abilities, appearance, intelligence, emotions, and interactions with other people. People with low self-esteem don't see themselves as valuable and underestimate their strengths and abilities; as a result, they are likely to lack self-confidence.

Although people talk about having low self-esteem or high self-esteem, many people have self-esteem that is midway between low- and high self-esteem and this "middle" or healthy self-esteem is thought to be the best for health and well being.

People with low self-esteem may not like or respect themselves. They may avoid new challenges or take dangerous risks in order to gain recognition or acceptance from their peers. People with low self-esteem let other people make choices and decisions for them because they often trust other people's ideas, reactions, and opinions more than their own. They often have unrealistic self-concepts, and focus more on their weaknesses and faults instead of seeing and appreciating their talents, abilities, and strengths.

People with low self-esteem are more bothered by failure and tend to exaggerate their own actions as well as actions of others as being negative. For example, they often make the mistake of taking comments that are not critical as criticism. They are more likely to be nervous and anxious around others, and they may feel awkward, shy, and unable to express themselves when relating to other people.

People with low self-esteem are more likely to be pessimistic about themselves and others. Instead of focusing on their goals for the future and achieving them, they are more likely to concentrate on not making mistakes. They are less likely to try new activities or challenge themselves.

Today, families always seem to be rushing. Everyone is busy with work, school, and other activities. Sometimes, even meals are hurried, and there is no time for family members to catch up with one another. Setting aside some time each week to sit down together and share thoughts, feelings, and plans can help families keep the lines of communication open. Communicating regularly helps families stay strong and close.

Research has shown that low self-esteem can harm health and well being. People with low self-esteem are more likely than people with middle or high self-esteem to neglect their health and treat themselves badly. They are less likely to take good care of themselves. They are more likely to eat unhealthy diets, overeat, abuse alcohol and drugs, and less likely to get enough exercise and practice good personal hygiene.

Teens with low self-esteem are less likely to do well in school and more likely to blame other people for their problems rather than taking responsibility for their actions. They are more likely to get into trouble for bad behavior at school and less likely to consider the needs of others.

Because people with low self-esteem crave approval and acceptance they tend to be "followers" rather than leaders and are more likely to be talked into participating in bad behaviors like skipping school or even criminal acts like shoplifting. Low self-esteem also has been linked to high-risk behaviors such as smoking, alcohol and drug use, unsafe sex, increased risk of developing eating disorders and teenage pregnancy.

On the other hand, it is important to realize that having low self-esteem does not mean that a person cannot live a happy, healthy, and successful life. Some people with low self-esteem strive to overcome their weaknesses and develop strengths or talents to compensate for their weaknesses. They may be very motivated to prove themselves. Not only can many people overcome their low self-esteem to achieve great success but by doing so they also may actually increase their self-esteem.

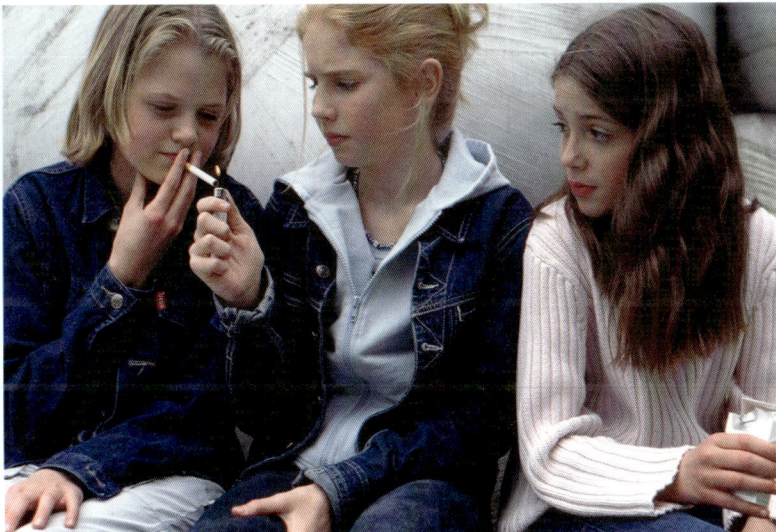

Those with low self-esteem are more likely to be "followers" who allow themselves to be pressured by friends, and studies have shown links between low self-esteem and risky behaviors like smoking. © DENISE HAGER/CATCHLIGHT VISUAL SERVICES/ALAMY.

Recognizing Low Self-Esteem

Sometimes it's easy to recognize when someone has low self-esteem. The person may be shy, insecure, withdrawn, unhappy, and unwilling to participate in school or other activities. But other times it's not as easy to recognize low self-esteem. There are common ways that a person who has low self-esteem might behave. The person with low self-esteem might act like:

Victims—Victims feel harmed and helpless to do anything about it. Instead of taking responsibility for their own actions and taking steps to change their situations, victims wait for someone to save or rescue them. They often whine and express self-pity. Victims tend to lean heavily on others, looking to them to make choices and decisions for them. They also want others to defend them. As a result they do not learn to make good decisions or stand up for themselves.

Rebels—Rebels act like they don't care what anyone thinks about them. They act as though the opinions of friends, parents, teachers, coaches, and others simply don't make any difference to them. To prove that they don't care what others think or say about them, rebels tend to blame other people, talk back and behave disrespectfully, break rules, and make fun of people who do follow rules.

Imposters—Imposters are putting on a show—they behave as though they are happy and carefree when they are actually insecure and afraid of failing. They are constantly worried that someone will find out that they are not as good, smart, or talented as they wish to be. Imposters tend to very self-critical and overly critical of others too.

Children and Teens with Low Self-Esteem

Most children have average or high self-esteem. Children who suffer from low self-esteem are often those who have not received enough love and support from their parents as well as children who often received physical punishment from their parents.

Other children may suffer from low self-esteem because they only receive positive attention from their parents when they behave or perform a certain way. For example, parents may seem only to care about the child when she gets a straight A report card or when he wins a soccer game. This kind of attention is called "conditional regard" because the child only gets the parents' attention under certain conditions.

Still other children may suffer from low self-esteem because they feel different from their peers. Children with physical disabilities or illnesses such as cancer and diabetes may lack confidence and have low self-esteem because their health prevents them from participating in some activities or doing as well as they would like. Children with learning disabilities also may have low self-esteem because they may compare their ability to learn with their classmates and peers who don't have learning problems.

Children with low self-esteem are not self-confident. They are insecure and tend to be shy, quiet, and withdrawn. They are often unhappy, and they don't communicate well. It's hard for them to have fun. Even though they may have friends, because they are insecure they may be more likely to give in to peer pressure to take risks, and they may be bullied.

Some children with low self-esteem may act angry and hostile. They may behave badly—bullying, cheating, and disobeying rules. Although all children misbehave at one time or another, a child who always behaves badly may be suffering from low self-esteem.

When children start school they may have a decrease in self-esteem because they do not have a sense of mastery of their new environment. They must learn to interact with teachers and peers in a new environment with new rules to follow. If they are unable to master learning as well as their classmates, their self-esteem may decrease. For example, children who cannot read by the end of second grade may feel they are not as smart or good as their peers who have learned to read.

Children who are challenged by learning or mastering athletic skills like throwing and catching a ball may suffer a loss of self-esteem. Those who have difficulty making friends and being accepted by their peers also may have lower self-esteem.

As children enter adolescence, self-esteem tends to fall. Experts believe that this decrease in self-esteem is caused by body image issues and other changes that occur during puberty such as changes in appearance, social changes, and hormonal changes. Teenage boys and girls become very concerned about how they look and how their peers view them.

As children, boys and girls tend to have similar levels of self-esteem but during the teen years, adolescent boys tend to have higher self-esteem than adolescent girls. A great deal of this difference is linked to body image issues and teen girls' concerns that they don't measure up to the models and celebrities they see in magazines, on television, and in the movies. Teenage girls with low self-esteem often have a poor or inaccurate body image. They are overly self-critical and may feel they are too fat or not pretty.

During adolescence self-esteem may be fragile—easily dropping in response to criticism from peers or friends, failing a test in school, being ignored by a friend, or not making a team. Teens with low self-esteem are especially likely to respond to events they consider failures because these failures reinforce their feelings that they are not worthwhile or good enough.

Healthy Self-Esteem

In general, self-esteem is highest when people see themselves as close to their ideal images of themselves—the people they want and strive to be. People with healthy self-esteem have realistic self-concepts—they see their strengths and weaknesses clearly and accurately. They value their skills, talents, and abilities and do not give too much

The National Association for Self-Esteem defines self-esteem as: "The experience of being capable of meeting life's challenges and being worthy of happiness." Self-esteem comes from living consciously and may be viewed as a person's realistic judgment of his or her abilities and worthiness.

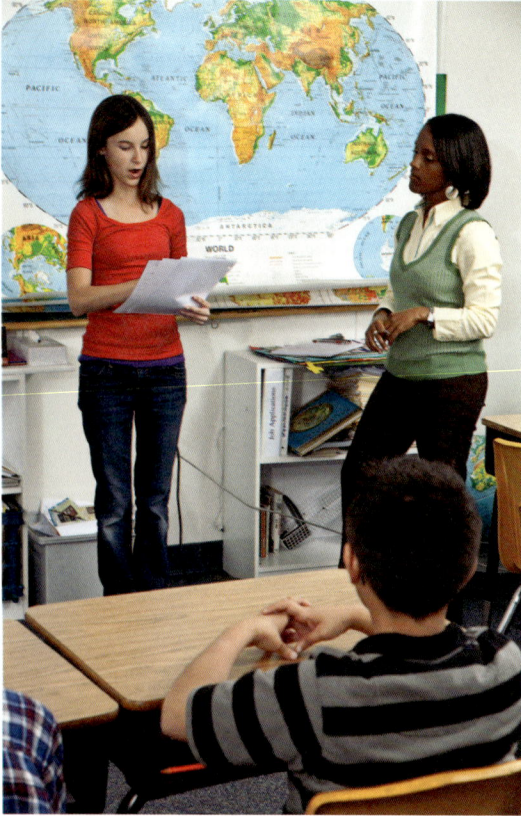

Giving presentations in the classroom in front of other students might be a little intimidating at first, but it is a good way to build up public speaking skills and bolster self-esteem. © MYRLEEN PEARSON/ALAMY.

importance to other people's criticism or negative impressions.

The National Association for Self-Esteem describes people with healthy or high self-esteem as those with "tolerance and respect for others, individuals who accept responsibility for their actions, have integrity, take pride in their accomplishments, are self-motivated, willing to take risks, capable of handling criticism, loving and lovable, seek the challenge and stimulation of worthwhile and demanding goals, and take command and control of their lives."

Healthy self-esteem is more than simply feeling good about oneself. It comes from a person's ability to set goals and work toward them, which in turn gives him or her a sense of satisfaction. Healthy self-esteem comes from knowing that one is generally capable of producing desired results, having confidence in one's ability to think, as well as to make appropriate choices and decisions. People with healthy self-esteem feel that they deserve to be happy.

Healthy self-esteem is genuine. It is based on good behaviors and actual effort and accomplishments. It is important that children, teens, and adults feel that they are "good enough" and worthy as long as these feelings are based on realistic self-concept. In other words, as long as their actions and behavior show that they really are good and worthy.

People with healthy high self-esteem are able to set realistic goals for themselves and take action to reach them. They have problems and setbacks in life, just as everyone does, but they do not let them interfere with their goals and plans. They view problems and setbacks as exceptions, not the rule, and they try to learn from constructive criticism.

Having healthy self-esteem is very important because it has an impact on every aspect of life. Self-esteem affects physical and emotional health, how well students do in school, whether people have satisfying relationships with families and friends, and the decisions they make throughout their lives.

Self-esteem is like health—you can have too little but you can't have too much. There is no such thing as too much healthy self-esteem.

Unhealthy High Self-Esteem

Some people confuse healthy self-esteem, which is genuine, with unhealthy high self-esteem, which is not genuine. Unhealthy high self-esteem may be the result of being praised when praise was not due or earned. For example, praising a child for "doing the best he or she could" when the child did not put forth any effort might produce false or unhealthy self-esteem. In fact, showering a child with undeserved praise and compliments actually may backfire because the child may then feel that no effort is needed to earn and receive praise.

People with unhealthy high self-esteem tend to be overly self-confident and act smug and superior to those around them. Rather than feeling that they are good enough, they feel they are better than everyone else. They may be selfish, self-centered, and assume that their needs and desires are more important than anyone else's. They also tend to overlook any of their own faults or weaknesses but are critical of others' weaknesses. Because they do not recognize their weaknesses they do not take steps to improve.

People with unhealthy high self-esteem often concentrate on specific qualities such as being attractive, popular, wealthy, or athletic. They focus on this quality and develop an undeserved, unrealistic, and exaggerated self-concept. This can lead to all kinds of bad behavior such as bragging, boasting, and showing off. They may try to boost their own feelings of self worth by bullying, insulting, and putting other people down.

Until recently, many experts thought that more self-esteem was always better than less self-esteem but it turns out that this isn't always true. Unhealthy high self-esteem can be just as harmful as low self-esteem. Children are as likely to behave selfishly if they are undervalued or overvalued. Research shows that people with unhealthy high self-esteem may have trouble controlling their impulses, are more likely to be bullies, and to participate in criminal activities and behaviors.

Friends Can Help or Harm Self-Esteem

Friends have a tremendous impact on a person's self-esteem. The quality of the friendships and how people spend time with their friends affects self-esteem. In general, if one's friends are positive, basically happy people with a healthy outlook on life then they will likely support one another and boost one another's self-esteem. On the other hand, if one's friends are pessimistic and spend most of their time together whining, complaining nonstop, and constantly criticizing one another they may be harming their self-esteem.

Healthy Friendships Boost Self-Esteem Healthy friendships are those in which the friends feel happy and support one another. Friends support and encourage one another to pursue dreams, goals, and ambitions.

Friends treat one another with respect and act like cheerleaders for one another and help to motivate one another to do well. Healthy friendships can improve teens' views of their peers and improve their peers' views of them.

In healthy friendships, friends praise and celebrate one another's achievements and accomplishments and encourage one another after failures because they are genuinely concerned about one another. In healthy friendships people feel a sense of belonging and community.

Friends are loyal—they stick up for one another. They listen to one another and help one another through hard times. They can encourage one another to avoid or change unhealthy habits like eating too much junk food and not getting enough exercise. They also can help one another cope with family problems, relationship problems, and other challenges. In healthy friendships, the friends feel accepted, trusted, cared about, and valued. Friends not only can support one another's self-esteem, they can actually boost it.

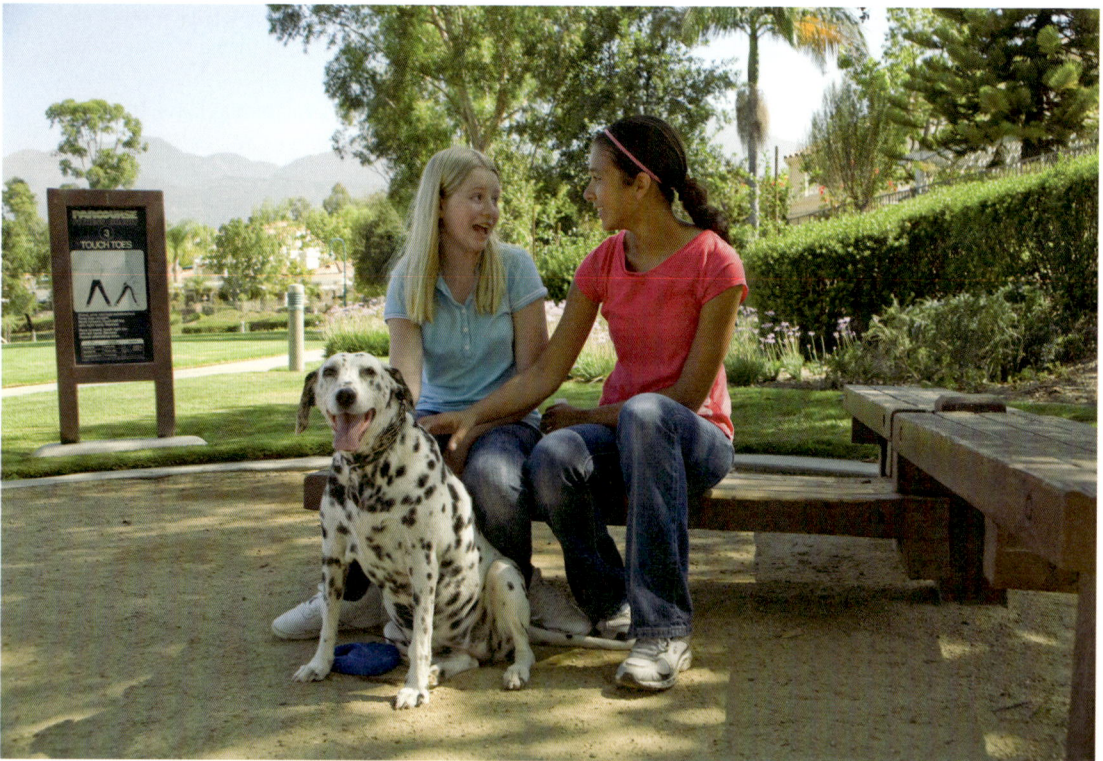

Friends sit and talk in the park. © MYRLEEN PEARSON/ALAMY.

Healthy friendships are not perfect. Friends in healthy relationships can disagree and even have conflicts. They are sometimes rivals and may at times behave badly toward one another. But because their relationship is based on trust, respect, and honesty, they can usually survive disagreements.

Unhealthy Friendships Harm Self-Esteem

Unhealthy friendships are those in which friends put one another down, take advantage of one another, and discourage one another from pursuing plans and goals. When friends are verbally abusive—making one another feel bad, discouraged, criticized, or belittled—the friendships are not healthy and do not support healthy self-esteem. People with negative outlooks on life and people who never see opportunities and only see problems are unable to support their own or others' self-esteem.

Friends who are not ambitious or who are afraid that they themselves will not be successful often try to discourage their friends' ambitions. They are especially likely to discourage others from trying to succeed or excel at activities in which they have been unsuccessful. For example, an unambitious person might discourage his friend from trying out for a team by saying, "Don't even bother to try out. I'm better than you are and I didn't make the team last year," or "Only losers want to be on that team." Surrounded by unambitious, unsupportive friends, it's easy for a person to lose sight of his or her own ambitions. When people lose sight of their ambitions, especially when they are young, it can limit their potential in life.

Finally, friends who often get into conflicts with one another, or who always try to dominate or assert their superiority over one another, are practicing a negative social behaviors that they

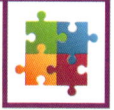

Making and Keeping Friends

Sometimes it's easy to make friends. People who share common interests like sports, chess, playing an instrument, or anime often become friends. Other times, like when a person enters a new school, it can be harder to make friends.

Making friends begins with smiling and saying "hi." Having a positive attitude and appearing open and friendly attracts people. Talking to people in class or after class is a good way to find out if they might be potential friends.

Ask people questions. Find out which teams they favor and ask about the music they like. It generally takes lots of introductions and greetings before people who will ultimately become friends meet and talk.

It's important for people to be the friends they want to make. People who are kind, considerate, and interested in others are more likely to attract good friends than scowling, rude, and inconsiderate people.

To keep healthy friendships, it's important to be a good friend. This means being trustworthy, keeping secrets and confidences, being a good listener, and offering advice only when friends ask for it. Friendships involve some back and forth—sometimes one friend gives encouragement and support, and other times he or she receives them. Treating friends with care, respect, and appreciation helps to maintain and strengthen friendships.

also may use with other peers and adults. These negative behaviors provoke negative reactions from friends, peers, and teachers. Those negative reactions encourage the students to become less and less involved with classmates and school, and to like school less. As a result they don't do well in school or in relationships with their peers, which in turn harms their self-esteem.

Avoid Actions and Behaviors That Harm Self-Esteem

Just as unhealthy friendships can harm self-esteem, there are other activities and actions that also may damage self-esteem. For example, it is important to choose a role model with healthy self-esteem. Young children with parents who are pessimistic, unrealistic, or very self-critical often copy this behavior and as a result do not develop healthy self-esteem. But as these children grow up, they can choose other role models, like a teachers or coaches, who have healthy self-esteem and copy their positive attitudes and behaviors.

It's equally important to learn to recognize and avoid abuse and abusive relationships. Abusive relationships with family members, friends, girlfriends, or boyfriends can seriously damage self-esteem. The most common types of abuse in teen relationships are emotional abuse, which is hurting someone's feelings on purpose; verbal abuse, such as name calling, threatening, bullying, or making fun of other people; and controlling behavior such as questioning people about their every move, telling them who they can see and who they should not see, or reading their e-mails and texts without their permission.

Know the warning signs of an abusive relationship. These are examples of signs that a relationship may be abusive.

- The person offers permission or says he or she will allow someone else to do something. For example, a boyfriend might tell his girlfriend, "You can have lunch with your friends today," or "I'll let you walk home from school by yourself tomorrow."
- The person monitors his or her friend's phone calls, texts, e-mail, and social networking Web sites like Facebook.
- The person tells his or her friend what to wear, how to act, and where to sit in class and the cafeteria.
- The person is jealous of other friends and becomes angry when he or she is not the center of attention.

Thomas Szasz (1920–2012), award-winning psychiatrist, author, and educator stated: "Every act of conscious learning requires the willingness to suffer an injury to one's self-esteem. That is why young children, before they are aware of their own self-importance, learn so easily."

- The person becomes angry frequently, has tantrums, and then blames others for his or her anger and tantrums.
- The person reacts to anyone with physical violence. A person who slaps, punches, or kicks someone is likely to do it again, even if he or she apologizes.

Violent Behavior

The Centers for Disease Control and Prevention (CDC) define violence as "use of physical force or power, against another person, group, or community, with the behavior likely to cause physical or psychological harm." Every year, about 700,000 youth ages 10 to 24 are treated in hospital emergency departments for violence-related injuries.

Examples of violent behavior include bullying, fighting, using weapons, gang violence, and electronic aggression, (also known as cyberbullying) which is "any type of harassment or bullying (teasing, telling lies, making fun of someone, making rude or comments, spreading rumors, or making threatening or aggressive comments) that occur through e-mail, a chat room, instant messaging, a Web site (including blogs), or text messaging."

A CDC survey finds that among high school students, about 6% said they did not go to school on one or more days in the 30 days before the survey because they felt unsafe at school or on their way to and from

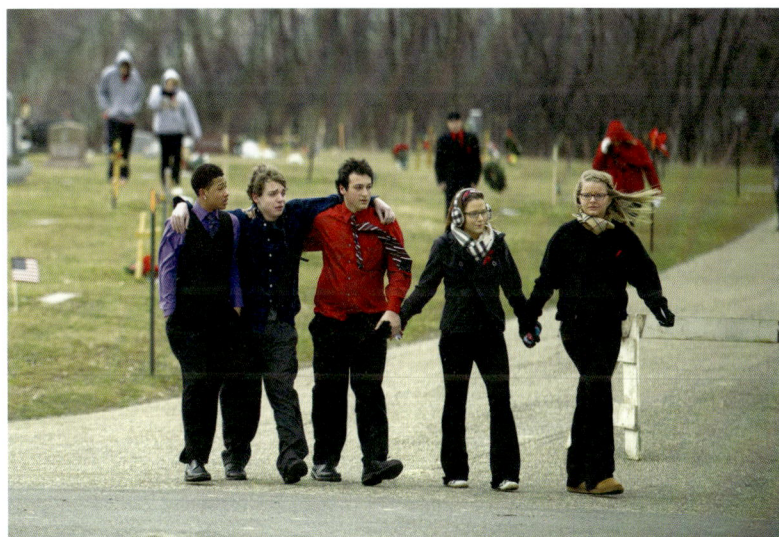

Mourners comfort each other as they leave the burial of Danny Parmertor at All Souls Cemetery on March 3, 2012, in Chardon, Ohio. Parmertor was killed by another student at Chardon High School in a shooting that left two other students dead and two injured.
© JEFF SWENSEN/GETTY IMAGES.

school. School violence can take place on school property, on the way to or from school, during a school-sponsored event, or on the way to or from a school-sponsored event.

Despite reports of violence on elementary school, middle school, high school, and college campuses such as the Columbine High School shooting in 1999 that claimed 13 lives and wounded 23 other people, the 2001 Santee, California, shooting that killed two students and wounded 13 others in 2001, the Red Lake, Minnesota, shooting that killed five students, a teacher, and security guard in 2005, and the Newton, Connecticut, shooting that killed 20 students and 6 adults in 2012, it is important to remember that most school campuses are safe. However, any violence on school campuses is unacceptable; students, parents, teachers, and administrators have a right to expect schools to be safe places, where students can learn and grow. School violence not only has a harmful effect on students but also on the community.

Bullying Bullying is when a person or group of people tries to harm someone who is weaker or someone they think is weaker. Sometimes bullying takes the form of physical attacks, but more often it involves threats, name-calling, teasing, taunting, or spreading ugly rumors.

Social bullying—telling other children or teens not to be friends with someone, leaving someone out on purpose to hurt his or her feelings, and embarrassing someone in public—can be just as hurtful as hitting, kicking, and punching.

Bullying is harmful. Children and teens that are bullied may feel so nervous and afraid that they avoid school. In the most serious cases, teens that are bullied may feel they need to run away or become violent with the person bullying them. Some become so depressed that they even consider suicide.

Although anyone can be bullied, some teens may be picked on more than others. Bullying is an aggressive form of prejudice, and bullies generally focus on people they think are different and unable to fight back. Throughout the United States, children are bullied because of their race, ethnicity, or religion; because they have disabilities; because they are smaller or shorter than their peers; or even because they are just somewhat shy and withdrawn. In some communities, lesbian, gay, bisexual, and transgender teens are at increased risk of being bullied.

Bullying can take place practically anywhere—at school, on the bus to and from school, at the playground or park, in the neighborhood, or even on the Internet. Bullying that takes place online or via text or e-mail using desktops, laptops, tablets, and cell phones is called cyberbullying.

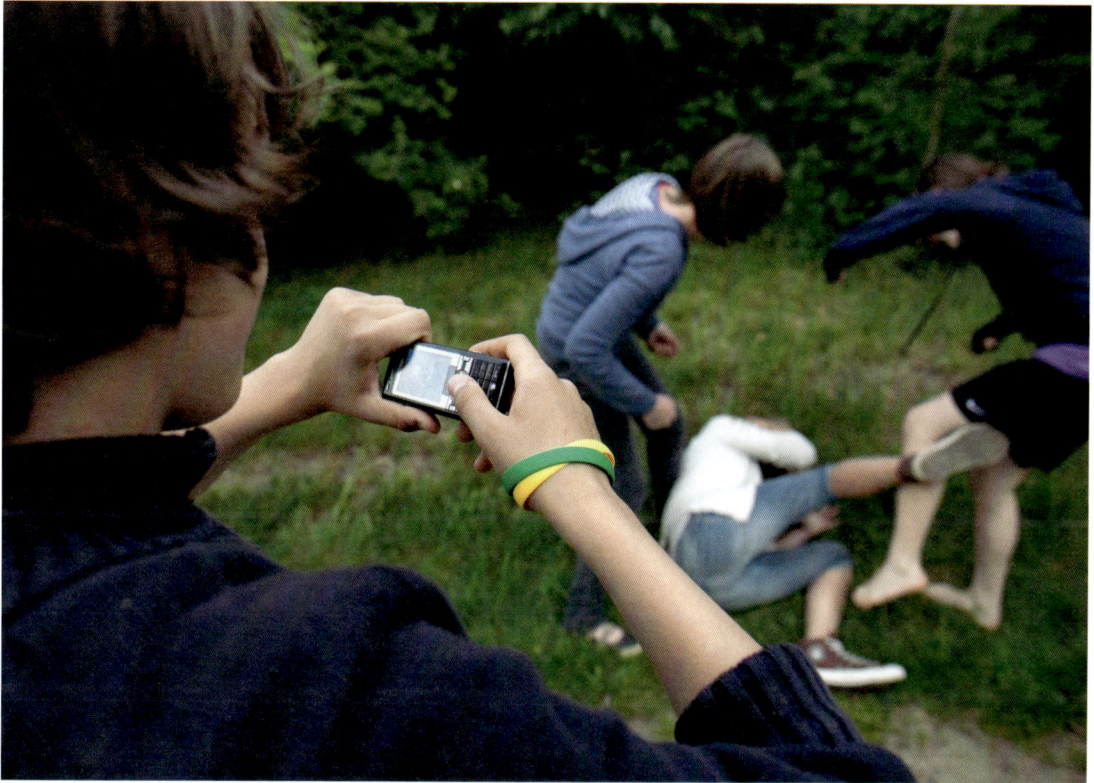

A teenage boy films girls bullying another girl on his mobile phone. © PHOTOTHEK/ANDIA/ALAMY.

Preventing and Responding to Bullying Unfortunately, some adults see bullying as "horseplay" and a normal part of growing up. They think that bullying should just be ignored. This is simply not true. When adults take immediate action to stop bullying, it sends a message to the school, team, community, and individuals that bullying will not be tolerated. Over time, this can help to prevent bullying.

It is important to tell a bully to stop. If this doesn't work, then it is best to simply walk away from the bully. When someone who has been bullied does not feel safe from the bully, he or she should try to stay near adults or groups of students.

If a person is bullied, or sees someone else being bullied, it is important to seek help immediately. Bullying should be reported to a trusted adult—a teacher, counselor, principal, coach, or parent. People who see someone being bullied should defend the person being bullied and help him or her to safely get away.

Cyberbullying Can Damage Self-Esteem Too

Cyberbullying—also called "electronic aggression,"—is a recent and very dangerous activity. It comprises the use of electronic devices and technology, the Internet, and social media sites to send mean or threatening text messages or e-mails, spread rumors by e-mail, or post embarrassing pictures, videos, Web sites, or fake profiles on social networking sites.

One of the reasons cyberbullying is so dangerous and harmful is because it is hard to escape it. A person can walk away from someone who is bullying him or her but cyberbullying can strike at any time of the day or night, and because messages and photographs may be posted anonymously, it may be difficult to identify and stop the cyberbullying.

Because young people who are cyberbullied are more likely to be afraid to go to school and skip school, they don't do as well as other students and may get bad grades. They also are more likely to use alcohol and drugs, have more health problems, and have lower self-esteem.

Although cyberbullying only really started with the widespread use of computers and cell phones, it is happening in cities, towns, and communities throughout the United States. Between 9% to 35% of young people in grades 6 through 12 report that they have been cyberbullied.

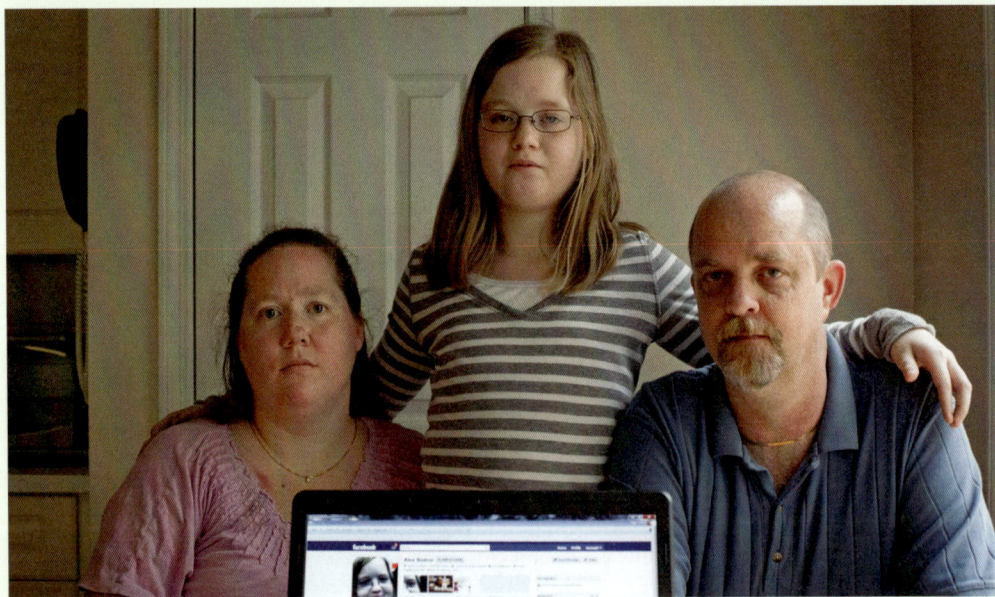

Alex Boston, 14, center, poses with her mother and father and a screen shot of the phony Facebook account that was set up in Alex's name. The family filed a libel lawsuit claiming two classmates humiliated Alex by using a doctored photo to set up the phony Facebook account in her name and then stacked the page with phony comments claiming Boston was sexually active, racist, and involved in drugs. © AP IMAGES/DAVID GOLDMAN.

Preventing School Violence Preventing school violence is everyone's responsibility. Many schools have school-wide or grade-specific programs aimed at reducing violent behavior between students. These programs help students improve their emotional self-awareness, emotional control, self-esteem, social skills, social problem solving, conflict resolution (the way to peacefully handle disagreements that threaten people's well being) and teamwork. Students that have learned these skills are better able to step in to stop violent behavior when it happens and to prevent it from increasing.

School-based programs also try to improve relationships between students and their peers, teachers, and families. When students and teachers have good relationships, students are more likely to feel comfortable going to teachers to talk about their fears or about violence-related issues.

Working with other violence prevention organizations, the CDC is using social media—Facebook and Twitter—to help prevent violence. People interested in violence prevention and leading safer, healthier lives can find articles, podcasts, and other violence prevention resources on Facebook at VetoViolence and Twitter. They also have the chance to interact with experts in real time, at events like a Twitter Live Chat about bullying prevention. The event took place during National Youth Violence Prevention Week in March 2012 and included experts from the CDC, the Anti-Defamation League, the U.S. Department of Education, and the Health Resources and Services Administration. The CDC reports that "during the live chat, #VetoViolence was one of the top 10 trending topics worldwide!"

Building Self-Esteem

Developing and maintaining a healthy, realistic self-concept and building self-esteem takes some work, but it is worth the effort. People with healthy self-esteem like themselves and value their health, so they take good care of themselves. They take pride in their health, safety, hygiene, and appearance.

There are many benefits of having healthy self-esteem. It helps people express their ideas, needs, and opinions confidently. It also helps them to develop secure and honest relationships. People with healthy self-esteem are less likely to try to please people at their own expense or to stay in unhealthy relationships.

Because they are happy with themselves, people with healthy self-esteem tend to get along well with other people and to behave responsibly. They also have more resilience—they can weather stress and recover from setbacks or illness more easily than people with low self-esteem. They also are better at facing and coping with unexpected challenges, disappointments, or illness.

It is perfectly natural for self-esteem to vary a bit from day to day. Everyone has days when everything seems to be going wrong; on days like these, self-esteem may suffer. Teenagers are especially prone to periods of self-doubt and concern about physical and emotional changes. Fortunately, these periods are usually brief, and the support of family, friends, teachers, and others can help teens over these rough patches.

There also are actions people can take to help support their own healthy self-esteem. These include:

Focusing on successes and accomplishments—taking pride in one's achievements and efforts boosts self-esteem. Instead of comparing oneself to others, it is more useful to look at one's own progress.

Judging oneself and others less often and less harshly—although self-esteem does involve an honest look at how one feels and values oneself, it is important to be realistic and not overly critical of oneself or others.

Setting realistic goals—Setting realistic standards for oneself and others makes it less likely that people will seek out flaws or weaknesses in themselves and others.

Asking others for help—To build self-esteem it may be helpful for teens to ask family and friends to describe the teen's strengths and the things he or she does do well. Go to teachers, guidance counselors, or tutors to ask for help in classes. To boost one's sense of competence, it may be helpful to learn a new skill like playing guitar or ice-skating. When these activities do not help to boost self-esteem, it may be helpful to talk with a counselor or therapist to explore feelings and learn ways to improve self-esteem.

Learning from mistakes—Everyone makes mistakes. Understanding that it is common to make mistakes helps people to be kinder toward themselves and others when things don't go as planned or mistakes are made. Mistakes can be viewed as valuable teaching lessons, helping people learn what not to do in a similar situation.

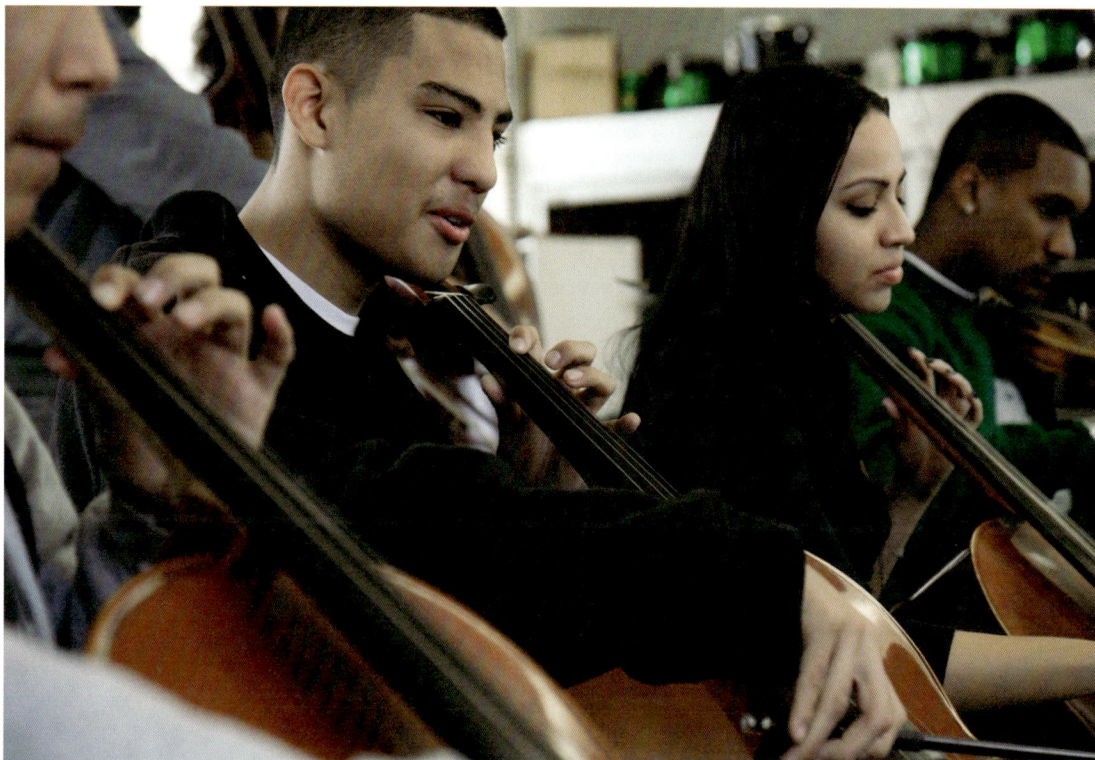

Focusing on the successes of skills already learned, like playing an instrument, or trying out a new skill can help boost self-esteem. © BLEND IMAGES/ALAMY.

Positive Self Talk Another important and useful way to support and maintain healthy self-esteem is by practicing positive self talk. Self talk is the term used to describe ongoing internal conversations people have with themselves, which influence how they feel and behave. A person's own thoughts can have a powerful effect on how they feel and on their self-esteem. Thoughts include "self talk"—what people tell themselves—how they look at events, people, and situations, and their beliefs about themselves and others.

People are always engaging in self talk even if they are entirely unaware of it. In order to change their self talk, people must become aware of it and identify self talk when it is happening. By noticing the messages and conversations, people can take stock of their self talk and use it to help them stay motivated, accomplish their aims, and maintain healthy self-esteem.

Positive self talk is optimistic and encouraging, it can help people take action, focus their energy, and become motivated. Athletes and other performers often use positive self talk to help them overcome obstacles to success such as exhaustion, physical pain and injury, or fierce competitors. Examples of positive self talk are, "I can do it" and "I am giving it my best effort" and "I know that anything is possible." Negative self talk, which everyone experiences from time to time is negative, discouraging, pessimistic, and critical. Examples of negative self talk are "Everyone in class is smarter than I am," "I am not good enough," and "I can't do it."

The body believes the self talk it hears. Self talk can create stress and make people nervous. For example, when preparing to make a speech in class, negative self talk, like, "I always freeze when I see my friends in the audience," or "I know I'll forget what I want to say when I get up in front of the class," actually causes physical changes in the body. The heart beats faster, breathing is shallow, and there may be a knot of tension in the stomach and sweaty palms. The rush of adrenaline, a hormone that is released during times of stress, may make it even harder to think clearly and feel confident.

Changing Negative Self Talk to Positive Self Talk Once people identify negative self talk there are steps they can take to stop it. One way to recognize negative self talk is to write down as much self talk as possible for a few days. By reviewing the self talk, it's pretty easy to see which self talk messages are positive and which ones are negative.

To stop negative self talk some people practice visualizing a stop sign or a red circle with a diagonal line through it. By holding up an imaginary stop sign when negative self talk appears, people can stop the negative message in its tracks. Getting rid of the nagging, nasty little voices that constantly put them down helps people improve their self-esteem and feel happier.

The next step is to replace negative self talk with positive self talk. To do this one has to be ready with positive messages to replace the negative self talk. Replace self-criticism with praise. Purposefully filling the mind with positive self talk leaves little or no room for negative messages.

Helping Others Boost Self-Esteem Helping other people in small ways, such as helping a neighbor carry groceries or joining an organized volunteer program, is a natural way to boost self-esteem. Giving one's time and energy to do a good deed, help someone out, or work for a worthy cause can help people to feel better about themselves and feel more positive and optimistic about the world around them.

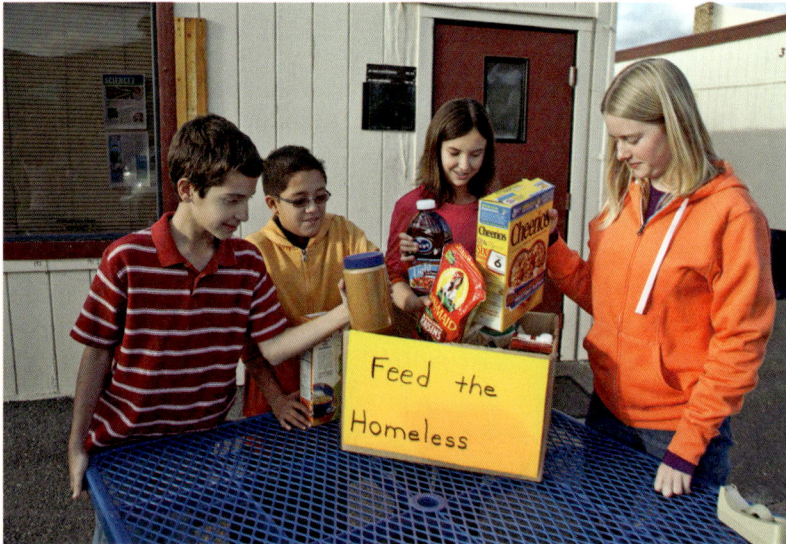

Volunteering is a terrific way to make new friends, learn new skills, and strengthen people's ties to the communities they live in. Whether it's working at a food bank, animal shelter, or peer-counseling program, volunteering has many benefits. Becoming a volunteer provides a healthy boost to self-confidence, self-esteem, and life satisfaction. By doing good for others and the community, people gain a genuine sense of accomplishment. Serving as a volunteer can also give people a sense of pride, purpose, and identity. When people feel better about themselves, they are more likely to feel motivated, optimistic, and happy.

Caring for Pets Boosts Health and Self-Esteem Pets are lots of fun, but their roles with humans go far beyond pure entertainment. They love to play, are nearly always happy to see their caregivers, and are loyal companions. Pets also are a big responsibility because they need plenty of attention as well as food, water, and exercise. But most pet owners agree that the benefits of having a pet make it worth all of the effort.

Caring for a pet has many health benefits. Children who have pets in their homes have fewer allergies and asthma, and some research has shown that pet owners make fewer visits to the doctor than people who don't have pets. One study found that children with pets missed fewer days of school than children without pets.

Pets can also help people get enough exercise and can even help to reduce stress and anxiety. Simply petting an animal's soft fur and feeling its warmth and heartbeat as it nuzzles or curls up close is soothing. Just being with a pet is calming and helps people feel happier.

Pets also teach people about unconditional love and about being gentle. Dogs and cats don't care what people wear or about their grades. Pets can help to strengthen family relationships and the bonds of friendship.

Children with pets in their homes also generally have healthier self-esteem and better social skills than children without pets. This may be because pets help to keep people from being lonely or because people and their pets depend on and support one another. It also may be that pets provide endless amusement and laughter with their unpredictable and often funny behaviors, keeping the mood of their human companions high.

For More Information

BOOKS

Capacchione, Lucia. *The Creative Journal for Teens: Making Friends with Yourself.* Franklin Plains, NJ: Career Press, 2002.

Fox, Marci, and Leslie Sokol. *Think Confident, Be Confident for Teens: A Cognitive Therapy Guide to Overcoming Self-Doubt and Creating Unshakable Self-Esteem.* Oakland, CA: Instant Help Books, 2011.

Lawrience, Michael. *Self-Esteem: A Teen's Guide for Girls.* Lawrience Publishing, 2012.

Palmer, Pat, and Melissa Alberti Froehner. *Teen Esteem: A Self-Direction Manual for Young Adults.* Atascadero, CA: Impact Publishers, Inc., 2010.

Schiraldi, Glenn. *The Self-Esteem Workbook.* Oakland, CA: New Harbinger Publications, 2001.

Zelinger, Laurie, and Jennifer Kalis. *A Smart Girl's Guide to Liking Herself, Even on the Bad Days.* Middleton, WI: American Girl, 2012.

WEB SITES

Hey U.G.L.Y. (Unique Gifted Lovable You): Empowering Youth to Be a Part of the Solution to Bullying. http://www.heyugly.org/ (accessed December 7, 2012).

National Association for Self-Esteem. http://www.self-esteem-nase.org (accessed December 7, 2012).

The Nemours Foundation. "TeensHealth: Body Image and Self-Esteem." http://kidshealth.org/teen/food_fitness/wellbeing/body_image.html (accessed December 7, 2012).

"A Positive Image: Self-esteem." *Palo Alto Medical Foundation*. http://www.pamf.org/teen/life/depression/selfesteem.html (accessed December 7, 2012).

"Teen Survival Guide: Bullying." *girlshealth.gov*. http://www.girlshealth.gov/bullying/ (accessed December 7, 2012).

"Teen Survival Guide: Self-Esteem." *girlshealth.gov*. http://www.girlshealth.gov/teenguide/feelinggood/index.cfm (accessed December 7, 2012).

"Ten Self-esteem Building Tips for Teens." *The Mental Health Association of South Central Kansas*. http://www.mhasck.org/news/article72.html (accessed December 7, 2012).

U.S. Substance Abuse and Mental Health Services Administration. "Building Self-esteem: A Self-Help Guide." https://store.samhsa.gov/shin/content//SMA-3715/SMA-3715.pdf (accessed December 7, 2012).

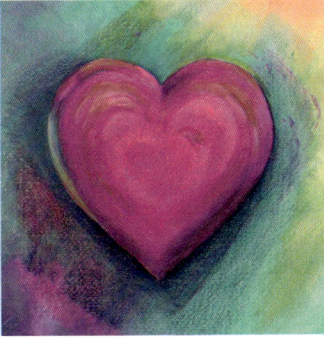

Mental Health

Introduction **435**

Nature vs. Nurture: How Do They Influence Development? **436**

Becoming an Individual: Personality, Individuality, and Temperament **440**

Memory **442**

Learning **444**

Intelligence **449**

Creativity **450**

Mental Health Therapies **452**

Psychotherapy **452**

Insight Therapy **452**

Cognitive and Behavior Therapies **461**

Pharmacotherapy **466**

Nontraditional Mental Health Therapy Techniques **467**

Therapy Formats **473**

Self-Help **480**

For More Information **480**

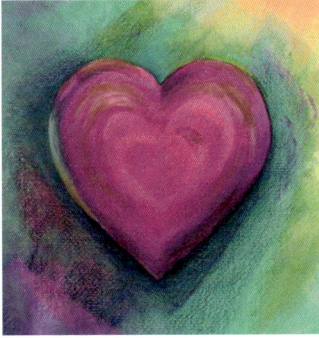

Mental Health

Mental health may be defined as a person's abilities to think and communicate clearly, learn and grow emotionally, cope with change and stress, and form and maintain good relationships with others. Mental health is linked to physical health and is an important part of wellness. Self-esteem, resilience, and the ability to cope with hardship influence how people feel about themselves and whether they choose lifestyles and behaviors that help or are dangerous for their health. While there is no one definition of ideal mental health, it is probably some combination of these characteristics along with a realistic view of the world and optimism.

Among the most studied questions in biology (the study of living organisms) and psychology (the study of the mind) is how the mind develops. How do people develop the capacity for learning, memory, intelligence, and personality? Why do two or more people, born to and reared by the same parents (and therefore possessing similar genetic makeup as their siblings), often turn out to have such different likes and dislikes, different strengths and weaknesses? Why do some people develop mental illness while their brothers or sisters do not?

There are different theories about how people develop and grow mentally and emotionally. Some experts believe that the environment in which a person is raised contributes not only to the development of personality but also to intelligence and can even foster or prevent the development of certain mental illness. Others believe that biology plays a bigger role than environment, and people develop in response to genetic programming. Today, most mental health researchers view both biological and environmental factors as important in the development and growth of the mind.

This chapter discusses different aspects of mental health, including identity and personality, memory, learning, intelligence, and creativity. Together, these areas are the qualities that make people who they are. It also describes mental health therapies and treatment for mental illness.

Words to Know

Art therapy: The use of art and craft activities to treat emotional, mental, and physical disabilities.

Bioenergetics: Body/mind therapy that aims to free the body and the mind of negative actions.

Biofeedback: The technique of teaching people to control involuntary bodily processes (such as heartbeats or brain waves).

Classic conditioning: Learning involving an automatic response to a certain stimulus that is acquired and reinforced through association.

Cognition: The mental processes of perception, recognition, conception, judgment, and reason.

Dance therapy: The use of dance and movement to treat or relieve symptoms associated with mental or physical illness.

Dream analysis: A technique of Freudian therapy that involves looking closely at dreams for symbolism and significance of themes and/or repressed thoughts.

Ego: The part of the personality that balances the drives of the id and the exterior world that is the center of the superego.

Existential therapy: Therapy that stresses the importance of existence and urges patients to take responsibility for their psychological existence and well-being.

Generativity: The ability or power to create, generate, or produce something.

Gestalt therapy: A humanistic therapy that urges individuals to satisfy growing needs, acknowledge previously unexpressed feelings, and reclaim facets of their personalities that have been denied.

Humanistic: A philosophy that places importance on human interests and dignity, stressing the individual over the religious or spiritual.

Hypnosis: A trance-like state of consciousness brought about by suggestions of relaxation, which is marked by increased suggestibility.

Id: According to Sigmund Freud, the biological instincts that revolve around pleasure, especially sexual and aggressive impulses.

Nature vs. Nurture: How Do They Influence Development?

The nature vs. nurture debate considers the following question: which factors contribute to mental development: nature (that is, the biological or genetic makeup of a person) or nurture (that is, how a person is raised, by whom, and in which environment). Just as human beings inherit certain physical traits from their biological parents (such as height, eye color, and even predisposition to physical ailments), they also inherit certain mental

Insight therapy: Therapy techniques that assume that a patients' behavior, thoughts, and emotions become disordered as a result of a lack of understanding of what motivates them.

Modeling: Learning based on modeling one's behavior on that of another person.

Music therapy: The use of music to treat or relieve symptoms of certain mental or physical illnesses.

Operant conditioning: Learning that involves voluntary response to a certain stimuli based on positive or negative consequences resulting from the response.

Pharmacotherapy: The use of medication to treat emotional and mental problems.

Psychiatry: The branch of medicine that relates to the study and treatment of mental illness.

Psychoanalysis: A theory of psychotherapy, based on the work of Sigmund Freud, involving dream analysis, free association, and different facets of the self (id, ego, superego).

Psychodrama: A therapy that involves a patient enacting or reenacting life situations in order to gain insight and change behavior. The patient is the actor while the therapist is the director.

Psychodynamics: The forces (emotional and mental) that develop in early childhood and how they affect behavior and mental well-being.

Psychology: The scientific study of mental processes and behaviors.

Psychotherapy: Treatment during which a trained mental health professional tries to help a patient resolve emotional and mental distress.

Rational-emotive behavior therapy: Therapy that seeks to identify a patient's irrational beliefs as the key to changing behavior rather than examining the cause of the conflict itself.

Reality therapy: A therapy that empowers people to make choices and control their destinies.

Stagnation: A state of inactivity; failing to grow, change, or develop.

Superego: According to Sigmund Freud, the part of one's personality that is concerned with social values and rules.

characteristics and traits from their parents, such as a tendency to develop certain mental disorders. Which traits and characteristics develop as a result of the environment in which a person is raised? Many researchers believe that intelligence and the tendency to develop diseases, such as alcoholism and other addictions, are largely inherited, while others argue that they are products of the environment in which a person is raised.

A mixture of nature and nurture is likely to determine individual traits and characteristics, including personality and behavior. Genetic factors may be viewed as the foundation on which environmental factors exert their influence. Today, it is widely accepted that while certain environmental factors alone and certain genetic factors alone may explain the origins of some traits and diseases, most of the time the interaction of both genetic and environmental factors is responsible.

In recent years, researchers have identified more and more genes that influence an individual's susceptibility to disease. Scientists have already linked specific DNA variations with increased risk of common diseases and conditions, including cancer, diabetes, hypertension, and Alzheimer disease (a progressive neurological disease that causes impaired thinking, memory, and behavior). These findings support the results of twin studies that show patterns of inheritance of mental health problems. Science in the 21st century recognizes genetic susceptibility but there is no support for the view that all persons carrying a specific genetic mutation will develop mental illness.

Intelligence The most controversial area in the nature vs. nurture debate is intelligence. The reason for this may be that intelligence (which is a person's capacity to learn, think rationally, and deal with challenges effectively) is closely related to achievement, in school and in other situations. Most researchers agree that intelligence is influenced by genetics to a great degree. Studies show that twins of all kinds and biological siblings are more likely to possess similar intelligence than those who are unrelated but raised together. In fact, the closer the biological link, the stronger the similarity in intelligence. However, there are also similarities in intelligence between unrelated children raised together in the same household, though these similarities are not as great as those between biological siblings and, especially, twins.

The exact way that genes and environmental factors interact to influence brain function, including intelligence, is still unknown. What is known is that a person's natural intelligence can be improved or obstructed by his or her environment.

Personality In addition to physical characteristics and intelligence, researchers look at how genetics and the environment influences personality. If a really outgoing, social person has a child, will that child also be outgoing? Some researchers say yes. In fact, scientists have been able to prove that personality types such as extroversion (being outgoing and social) and neuroticism (being touchy, moody, or overly sensitive) are often inherited.

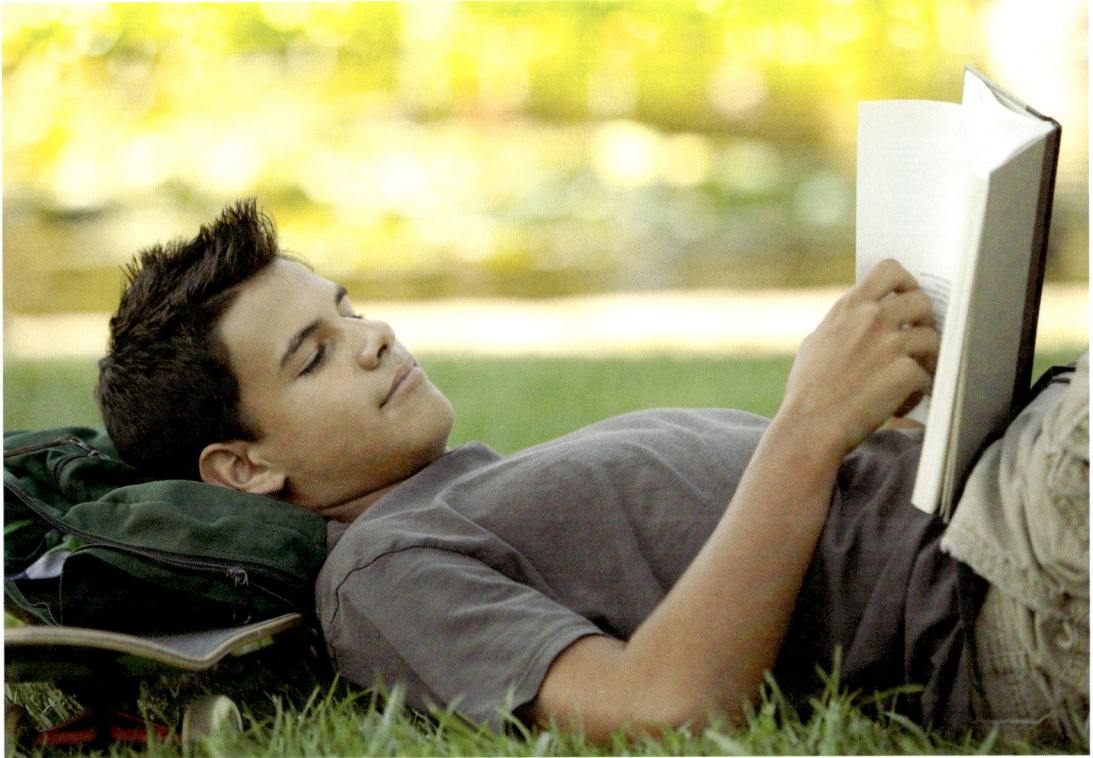

Though intelligence is thought to be inherited to some extent, environmental factors also influence intelligence. Developing good study habits, such as reading daily, helps develop good thinking and reasoning skills. © PHASE4PHOTOGRAPHY/SHUTTERSTOCK.COM.

Twins are useful for these studies because nearly all twins share the same home environment, but only identical twins share exactly the same genetics. Studies involving twins living apart have found that many qualities and characteristics seem to be inherited—from values and political attitudes to the amount of time people spend watching television! This may sound silly and, of course, no one is suggesting that a specific gene has evolved that directly influences a person's preference for watching television. Rather, researchers focus on the fact that watching television is often a solitary, passive activity. This could be related to whether a person is introverted or extroverted.

Other genetic links to personality and behavior have been discovered, such as the tendency for risk-taking—some people enjoy taking risks like bungee jumping or extreme sports, while others do not. Researchers also find that genetics strongly influence on people's sense of self-control and their social and learning abilities as well as their sense of purpose.

Most researchers agree that biology and environment play important roles in shaping people. Just as children may share traits with biological parents, adopted children also share many traits and habits with their adoptive parents. One theory proposes that genes probably influence tendencies or natural inclinations, which then are shaped by environmental experiences in ways that increase the likelihood of the individual developing specific traits and attitudes. For example, children or teens that are small for their ages might be teased by their larger peers. As a result, they might develop anxieties about social interactions, which might then influence their personalities. They might become shy, have low self-esteem, and develop attitudes such as a dislike of large groups.

Becoming an Individual: Personality, Individuality, and Temperament

Each person has a unique combination of behavioral traits, feelings, likes and dislikes, and habits. This special mix is called personality. Heredity, environment, and behavior determine and then shape personality throughout life.

Personality Personality is the sum total of the physical, mental, emotional, and social characteristics of an individual. It is the quality that makes each person unique. There are several basic personality types and many variations of each type. For example, some people are extroverted (outgoing), some are introverted (shy, reserved) and many people are somewhere in between. Some people are optimistic (positive) while others tend to be more negative, seeing the downside of situations rather than the upside.

The type of personality a person has may, according to mental health professionals, cause him or her to seek out situations that agree with his or her view of the world and personality. This results in a certain consistency, in which the personality drives choices and decisions that reinforce a person's personality.

Individuality As personality begins to develop, it is reinforced and solidified during adolescence when young people begin to ask, "Who am I?". This quest for individuality is perhaps best illustrated by looking at the work of renowned psychoanalytic theorist Erik Erikson (1902–1994), who mapped out an eight-stage process that covers all stages of development, with the stages in adolescence focusing on identity and individuality.

Erikson's stages include stage one, basic "trust versus mistrust," which takes place in infancy and centers on an infant learning trust by being cared for properly. During the toddler years, stage two, the "autonomy (independence) versus shame and doubt" stage, is resolved by allowing children to assert their independence and not feel bad for misbehaving or failing at their attempts at independence such as "accidents" during toilet training.

Stage three consists of a conflict related to "initiative versus guilt" in early childhood; at this time children begin to act on curiosities and explore new things, and the conflict is resolved if children are encouraged in their new interests and curiosities. In middle childhood stage four emerges, involving "industry versus inferiority;" during this stage a child must acquire skills in order to avoid feeling inferior (less worthy than others).

Stage five, a pivotal stage in terms of this discussion, involves "identity versus role confusion" in the teen years. During this time, adolescents try to form their own personal identities based on their childhood identities and where they wish to go—personally and professionally—in the future. Teens that prematurely set themselves in a certain identity are at risk for having grasped onto identities that are largely based on the approval of friends. Teens that do this may be less autonomous (independent) and inquisitive (eager to learn) than others. They may grow up to be people who are not open to change and new experiences.

Another problem that can arise during the fifth stage of development is identity confusion—teens who simply are never really certain about who they are and their place in the world. People suffering from identity confusion run the risk of being unable to forge meaningful relationships, in part because of their immature behavior and reasoning.

For all of these reasons, it is very important that children and young adults be encouraged to figure out their likes and dislikes, talents and natural inclinations, and to try new things during the development process so that they will develop a sense of identity.

Stage six is concerned with the conflict of "intimacy versus isolation" during early adulthood. During this time, people seek out deep, meaningful intimate relationships or choose to isolate themselves, possibly with very negative consequences later in life. Stage seven presents a conflict of "generativity (growth or creativity) versus stagnation," meaning that people should feel that they have contributed to the development of other people, particularly young people, or they will be left feeling the effects of stagnation (not changing or growing), which is the opposite of generativity.

The last stage, stage eight, "ego integrity versus despair," occurs in late adulthood. At this stage, adults reflect on the lives they have led, their accomplishments and choices, and whether they have contributed to the betterment of society.

Memory

Memory is one of the most important functions of the brain. Memories define people and shape their identities. Without them, people would not know where they came from, what they have experienced, or the identities of their families and friends. Memories are unique to each person. While many people may witness or experience the same event, each person will understand and remember it differently. This is why memory is considered part of a person's complex personality.

Scientists know what memory is, but they still don't know exactly how it works. Memory is defined as the ability to acquire information, store it, and then retrieve it later. It affects every aspect of people's daily lives. People remember facts, such as their names, phone numbers, and birth dates. They also have memories of past events, such as graduation from high school, getting married, or the death of a loved one. In addition, people have memories of certain skills, such as how to talk, walk, cook, or play a sport. Still other memories seem to be instinctive. For example, people remember how to sleep, breathe, and digest food. Memory helps people learn and live.

Different Kinds of Memory Types of memory fall into two categories, or systems, in the brain. One system deals with factual knowledge, such as names and dates. The other system deals with skills.

Factual knowledge is usually referred to as short-term memory. Short-term memories can become long-term if the circumstances are right. Scientists are still unclear as to exactly how this works; however, they think that short-term memories do not last long because new information enters the part of the brain that stores short-term memories and then drives out older memories. If a short-term memory passes into the long-term memory, it has more staying power. It lasts longer and may eventually become permanent. The longer a memory lasts, the stronger it is and the less likely it will be forgotten. This happens because short-term memories are fragile, while long-term memories are sturdier. Some scientists believe that long-term memories are stored permanently because of chemical changes in the brain.

Other scientists think that the length of a memory depends on certain circumstances; however, they do not know which circumstances produce long-term memories and which produce short-term memories. One thing scientists agree on, however, is that the brain seems to have an unlimited capacity to store memories. Scientists continue to study how people store and retrieve memories. One question that as yet remains unanswered is "If people have an unlimited capacity to remember information, why do they forget some things?"

How People Remember and Why They Forget

When memories are stored in the brain, they cannot serve people unless they are retrieved. How do people retrieve memories? This usually happens when memories are challenged. For example, if someone asks a question, a person must attempt to retrieve information in order to answer the question. Sometimes the answer is easy; other times, a person takes time to answer it. The amount of time it takes to answer the question is connected to a person's awareness of which memories are stored. Sometimes people are not aware at the time that they know the answers, but later realize that the information is there, ready to

Ways to Improve Memory

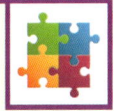

The capacity to store information long-term is connected to concentration. Short-term memories can easily become long-term if a person is willing to concentrate on the facts. Lynn Stern, author of *Improving Your Memory,* says that to make a long-term memory a person must "focus on it exclusively for a minimum of eight seconds." With training, anyone can improve the capacity to remember.

Other ways to improve and maintain a good memory are to:

- Exercise on a regular basis. Exercise helps keep the blood flowing, which increases the amount of oxygen that reaches the brain. With more oxygen, the brain, and therefore the memory, stays sharp and focused.

- Manage stress. Stress can affect the body and the mind in negative ways. Emotional disorders such as depression can harm a person's ability to retrieve information.

- Stay organized. Organization creates order in a person's life. If a person is always losing her keys, her brain is being used to try to find them every day instead of thinking about more important matters.

- Use visualization. Visualization means creating an image that corresponds with a fact or an event. If a person is trying to remember a list of groceries, it is helpful to associate a word, such as bread, with its corresponding image.

- Write it down. Writing things down on paper or typing them onto a computer, netbook, pad, or smart phone helps people to remember because the act forces them to concentrate on the things they are writing.

be retrieved. Sometimes, a smell or a sound can trigger a memory that a person did not know was there.

Retrieving a memory involves finding the path that leads to the information and navigating that path. As more and more memories are stored from new experiences, those paths can become intertwined, making it more difficult to find the way back. It can become particularly difficult when stored information has similar meaning because a person may have trouble distinguishing between memories. For example, if a person has seen hundreds of movies, it may be difficult to recall the details of each one. The person may mix together certain parts or lines from different movies or may even confuse the actors involved in the movies.

Some people have trouble retrieving a memory, but eventually manage to do it. However, sometimes a memory cannot be retrieved at all. Does this mean that the information has disappeared forever? Scientists believe that as people search for a particular memory, such as the name of a childhood friend for example, they are actively retracing the path to find the original information that was stored years ago. If they make it there, the memory is retrieved. However, if people cannot seem to make it back on that path, they will never be able to find the memory. Sometimes, though, people will find their way by taking an alternate route. For example, if a person asks a friend a question, and the friend thinks he knows the answer but cannot seem to retrieve the information, he might say something like, "It's on the tip of my tongue!" Then, as he is doing something completely unrelated later in the day, the information might pop into his head. Scientists believe this happens because the brain has found a related item, which then helps the person find the desired information.

Learning

When most people think of learning, they think of acquiring knowledge or a specific skill, such as facts about history, new vocabulary words, or how to play an instrument. Learning also encompasses behavior in a much broader sense. To mental health professionals, learning involves behavior modification. For example, when students learn how to do long math problems, they use a process that a teacher showed them, but they are actually learning a behavior (how to solve long math problems). As a result, when presented with a math problem in the future, they can draw on that behavior (or learned method) to solve the problem.

Of course, not everything that people do is learned through teaching or firsthand experience. Some behaviors are purely instinctual, behaviors that people (and animals, too) are genetically programmed to exhibit in certain situations. An example of this is the fight-or-flight impulse. In a scary situation, the human body produces adrenaline, which makes the heart pump faster and the lungs work harder. This is an unconscious response that readies a person to "fight" if the situation calls for it or to "flee"; this is not a learned response to fear or danger, it is an instinctual (a natural or innate impulse, inclination or tendency) one.

The Biology of Learning When babies are born, their brains are made up of billions of neurons (nerve cells that carry messages to and from the brain to other parts of the body). Over time, connections called synapses form between the neurons that are vital for proper brain functioning. These synapses help people make mental connections between different areas of the brain and between different information so that they may learn and develop to their fullest mental abilities. Stimulation, particularly during infancy and early childhood, drives the establishment of these synapses. Stimulation is anything that captures children's attention and makes them think, which can be anything from color, to light, sound, or touch. When stimulation occurs, synapses are built and strengthened. Without stimulation or even reinforced stimulation, key synapses either will not form at all or will wither away. While qualities such as intelligence and creativity may be largely influenced by heredity, these connections determine their maximum development.

Helping and Hindering Learning Stimulation is vitally important to help people realize their cognitive potential. Because the most important connections are made before the age of 10, it is important for children to receive proper stimulation. The key to optimizing learning and mental development for children includes:

- A nurturing, secure environment that provides emotional caring and safety.
- A sense of predictability so that children develop a sense of emotional stability.
- Conversation and communication; the spoken word boosts brainpower.
- Encouragement and praise of a children's accomplishments, to provide a sense of mastery and empowerment.

- Helping children make cognitive connections by pointing them out. (For example, pointing out a car in a picture and then taking the child for a ride in the car.)
- Knowing when a child has had enough stimulation and needs some quiet time.

Although learning problems such as attention-deficit disorder and other learning disabilities can hinder learning, certain environmental factors and conditions also may hurt a child's ability to learn. A neglectful home environment in which stimulation is absent can spell the beginning of future learning problems for a child. Particularly stressful events, such as the death of a parent, or a stressful situation, such as homelessness, also may have unfavorable effects on a child's ability to concentrate on and respond to mental stimulation.

Kinds of Learning Several kinds of learning occur throughout life that influence the acquisition of knowledge and changes in behavior. Proposed by prominent doctors, scientists, and therapists throughout the years, their principles remain unchanged and are the foundation for many forms of therapies.

Classical Conditioning. Formulated by Russian physiologist Ivan Pavlov (1849–1936), classical conditioning involves an automatic response to a particular stimulus that is acquired and reinforced through association. Pavlov illustrated the principles of classical conditioning after training dogs to salivate (involuntarily) upon hearing the ringing of a bell. He accomplished this task by first ringing a bell just before he fed the dogs. After a while, the dogs began to associate the ringing of the bell with dinner. However, the response was ingrained in the dogs on such a deep level that the food was no longer the stimulus for salivation; rather, the ringing of the bell alone made the dogs salivate.

This can be seen in people's everyday behavior in different situations. An infant will learn to respond to the sound and smell of its mother before being nursed or given a bottle; the child is responding not to the nutrients, but to the voice or scent of the mother. Similarly, if every time a child's parent calls him by his full name ("Come here, John Michael Smith!"), he is punished, his heart may beat faster just hearing his full name called, before his parent has even scolded him.

Operant Conditioning. Unlike classical conditioning (which involves involuntary response to a certain stimuli), operant conditioning

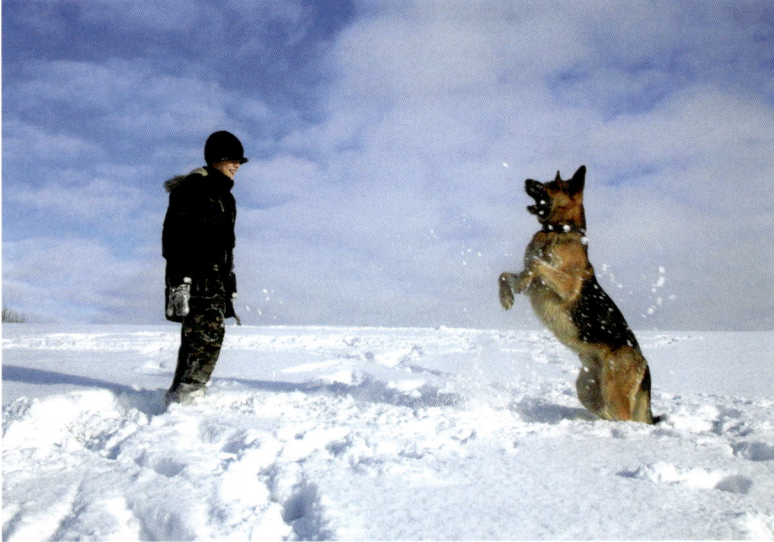

Operant conditioning can be used in dog training, for example by giving a dog a treat when it performs a wanted behavior. This desired behavior then becomes positively associated with a reward.
© KATARZYNA MAZUROWSKA/ SHUTTERSTOCK.COM.

involves voluntary response to a particular stimulus based on positive or negative consequences that result from the response. First put forth by psychologist B. F. Skinner (1904–1990), an example of operant conditioning is training a dog by using treats or verbal praise to reinforce behavior. If an owner trains her dog Fido to give her a paw when the dog's shoulder is touched, and the dog performs the task and is rewarded with a biscuit or kind words, the dog will associate successfully performing the task with the tasty treat or praise. Similarly, if a dog is consistently scolded when it chews something it should not, the dog will make the association between chewing a forbidden item with harsh words and will learn not to engage in that behavior. The same principles apply to human behavior. If a child learns that she is rewarded by successfully completing her homework each night, doing her homework will become important to her.

Positive reinforcement of a behavior will usually cause that behavior to continue, while punishment or the absence of reinforcement will result in ending the behavior. Behavior modification, a way of promoting positive behavior and eliminating negative behavior, is based on the principles of operant conditioning.

Observational Learning. Another way that people learn is by watching others or observing. A teacher showing students how to add several numbers together will often explain the principles behind the method and will then demonstrate the method by solving a sample problem. The students learn by observing the teacher. This is true of sports as well (watching a team execute certain plays during a sporting event) or behavior (watching someone get a desired result by giving a certain response). For example, a person might learn how to disarm her parents when they are angry with her by observing and adopting her brother's response, which seems to effectively calm their parents.

Observational learning is important in social learning. Young adults are likely to observe the habits and behaviors of their peers and adopt them as their own if they see their peers gaining social acceptance through those habits and behaviors. The behaviors adopted may be harmless, such as ways of dressing or taste in music, or harmful, such as choosing to smoke or take drugs.

Modeling (basing one's behavior on that of another person with whom there is a strong identification or desire to be like) is part of observational learning, and young adults often model their friends' behavior. Modeling can also take place between people they admire but do not personally know, such as a celebrity. For instance, if a young adult is a fan of Lady Gaga and hears that she does yoga every day, that young adult might take up yoga. The same holds true even if the person upon whom the teens are modeling themselves engages in harmful

A father explains a smoke detector to his daughters, demonstrating both observational learning, by showing them how to work it, and modeling, by exhibiting behavior that teaches responsibility and safety.
© JOCHEN TACK/ALAMY.

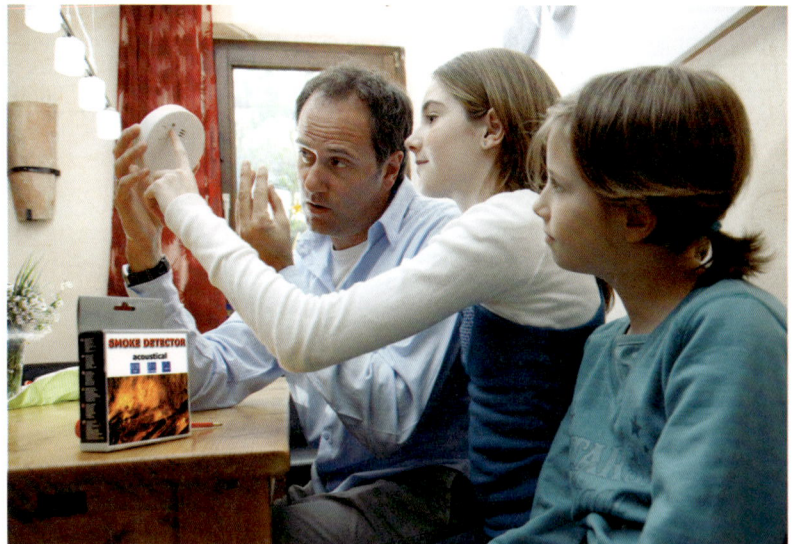

Healthy Living, 2nd Edition

behavior. A celebrity caught engaging in risky behavior may influence young adults (and older adults) to engage in similar behaviors. Celebrities and public figures are often called "role models," even when they do not wish to be. They are generally held to higher standards than other people because their behavior is more likely to influence a large number of people.

Intelligence

Intelligence is broadly defined as the ability and capacity to understand. To understand differences between very intellectual individuals and those who are less so Alfred Binet (1857–1911), a French psychologist, looked at why some students in French schools in the early 20th century were not learning at the same pace as other students. Using a trial-and-error approach to design an intelligence test, Binet developed questions based on a division of students into categories of "bright" or "dull." The questions that ended up on the test were the ones that reinforced the difference in knowledge between these two groups.

The intelligence quotient (IQ) is a measure of intelligence as based on intelligence tests and compared to the intelligence of the general population. While Binet created and published the very first standardized test of human intelligence (which was revised several times), it was American psychology professor Lewis Terman, of Stanford University, who came up with the actual formula for determining IQ: divide the test taker's "mental age," which is revealed by his or her score on the intelligence test, by his or her chronological age. The resulting number is what Terman called the intelligence quotient or IQ. In 1916 Terman brought the existing Binet test from France to the United States, translated it into English, and developed a new set of standard questions for American children. He named the new test Stanford-Binet.

In the general population the average IQ is 100. About two-thirds of people have IQs ranging between 85 and 115. People with IQs between 115 and 130 are classified as having superior IQs while those with IQs over 130 are labeled as gifted. People with IQs below 85 are labeled as borderline and any score under 70 often indicates that an individual is mentally impaired to some degree.

IQ tests have come to be viewed as predictors of a person's performance in school and in many careers. Over the years, however, the idea of intelligence, which is strongly tied to Binet's initial test, has come under fire. The notion of intelligence and ways of measuring it do not take into account that people with learning disorders may be very intelligent but may have trouble with the standard test. In addition, intelligence tests are culturally biased (preferential to certain groups of people) and may favor one group over another.

For example, the Stanford-Binet Intelligence Scale includes questions for young children about "typical" daily activities. However, depending on where children live—in the city or in the country or in California or New York—their typical experiences may be quite different, and it may be difficult for some children to come up with the "correct" answers. In the case of adult testing, participants are asked to interpret the meaning of "common" proverbs (short sayings such as "A stitch in time saves nine"). It may be difficult to answer these questions correctly if people have never heard the proverb, or if the proverb has a slightly different meaning depending on where a person grew up. Is it fair to say that someone possesses less intelligence than someone else because his or her life experiences do not coincide with the intelligence test?

Critics of this type of intelligence testing propose that basic intelligence is not necessarily tied to knowledge, the acquiring of which has cultural biases. These concerns have given rise to a variety of intelligence tests that are less culturally biased and measure not only verbal skills but also nonverbal skills.

Creativity

While intelligence refers to the capacity to understand, creativity is the capacity to think in unique ways and solve problems in an imaginative manner. Intelligence and creativity are not necessarily linked. People who are highly intelligent may not be very creative at all, while extremely creative individuals may not have a particularly high IQ. Creativity can be demonstrated in many ways, from creative writing to painting to architecture to simply performing a task in a creative manner, whether it is parenting, teaching, or building and repairing things.

Creative Thinking The key to creativity lies in divergent (different) thinking. Many people respond to questions using convergent thinking (thinking that is driven by knowledge and logic). Divergent thinkers respond to queries with unusual but still appropriate answers. For example, if a convergent thinker was asked how many ways he could think of to use a book, he might respond with a conventional answer such as, "You can read it and learn from it." A divergent thinker also gives conventional answers such as those given

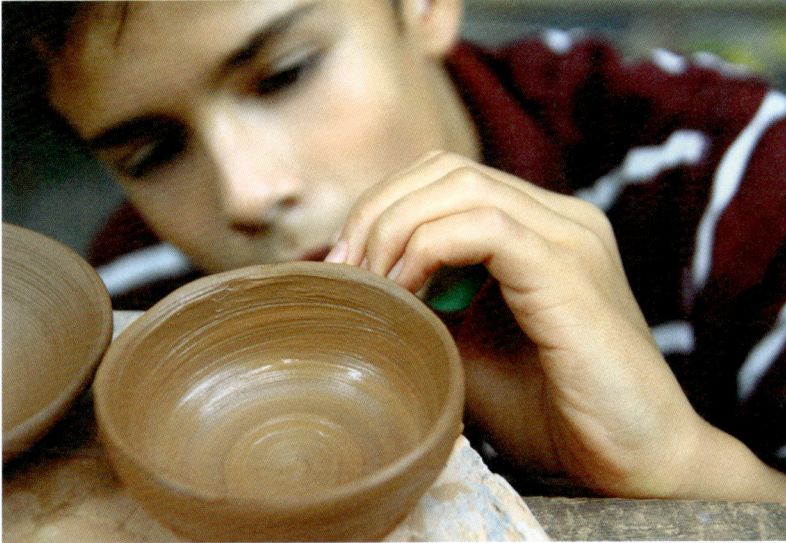

by a convergent thinker. But she may be more creative and say, "You could pile books on top of each other to create a step stool, or you could use the book as a doorstop, or you could use it as a serving tray."

Creative people tend to share certain characteristics, including a tendency to be more impulsive (spontaneous) than others. Nonconformity (not going along with the majority) can also be a sign of creativity. Many creative people are naturally unafraid of experimenting with new things; furthermore, creative people are often less susceptible to peer pressure, perhaps because they also tend to be self-reliant and unafraid to voice their true feelings even if they go against conventional wisdom.

How to Promote Creativity Child development specialists suggest that there are specific ways to promote creativity in children. Parents, caregivers, and teachers can encourage children to think divergently and come up with many different answers to a question or problem, answers that may fall outside of a traditional response. Adults should be careful not to ridicule an offbeat solution; rather, this sort of response should be taken seriously. Children should be encouraged to be free thinkers who do not always accept things as they are but, rather, question what is and why it is. In this vein, too, kids should feel they have a right to examine things independently and not always accept the answer, "Because that's just the way things are."

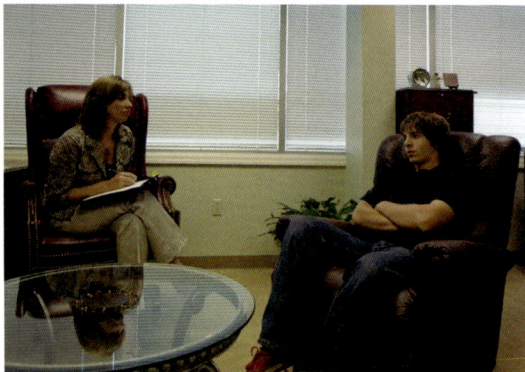

A teenager sits through a session with a psychotherapist.
© EIGHT ARTS PHOTOGRAPHY/ ALAMY.

There is a wide range of services, therapies, and therapists available to help persons suffering from mental illness. Mental disorders and mental health problems may be treated by highly trained medical and mental health professionals, as well as a variety of skilled practitioners from other disciplines such as pastoral counselors, school guidance counselors, child welfare specialists, and peer counselors.

Although none of these activities guarantees that a child, teen, or adult will necessarily be a creative person, it will help people to think creatively and to "color outside the lines."

Mental Health Therapies

Over time, mental health treatment in the United States—attitudes about, and care for, persons suffering from mental illness—has undergone many changes. This section describes the types of treatment used today and efforts to provide the most appropriate, and ideally most effective treatment, for each patient.

Psychotherapy

Psychotherapy is the general term for "talk therapy" with trained mental health professionals. Talking about problems with mental health professionals can help many people better understand their feelings. The success of the patient-therapist relationship relies on a good match between an informed, understanding, sensitive therapist; mutual trust; and the shared goal of changing destructive, unhealthy, or negative thoughts, attitudes, emotions, and behaviors. Psychotherapy aims to identify and resolve conflicts, increase self-awareness, and improve problem solving and communication skills.

Psychotherapy is used to treat a wide variety of conditions such as depression, anxiety disorders, and eating disorders. It is often used in combination with drug therapy. Some people respond well to psychotherapy, and some do well with drug treatment. Others do best with a combination of treatment—drugs and therapy.

Insight Therapy

Insight therapy assumes that a people's behavior, thoughts, and emotions become disordered because they do not understand what motivates them, especially when a conflict develops between their needs and drives. Insight therapy is based on the idea that a greater awareness of motivation will improve control and an improvement in thought, emotion, and behavior. The goal of this therapy is to help people discover the reasons and motivation for their behavior, feelings, and thinking. There are different types of insight therapy and several of these are described below.

Psychoanalysis Labeled by some as the "Father of Psychoanalysis," Sigmund Freud (1856–1939) introduced psychoanalysis, therapy based on the idea that psychopathology (the study of the nature and development of mental disorders) is a result of "unconscious conflicts" within a person.

Freud believed that personal development is based on inborn, and particularly sexual, drives that exist in everyone. He also believed that the mind, which he termed the psyche, is divided into three parts. These three parts of the psyche work together in a relationship called psychodynamics.

The Id. The id is the part of the mind in charge of all the energy needed to "run" the psyche. It governs unconscious urges and impulses like the basic biological urges for food, water, elimination, warmth, affection, and sex. The id works on immediate gratification and operates on what Freud called the pleasure principle: it aims to rid the psyche of developing tension by using the pleasure principle, which is the tendency to avoid or reduce pain and obtain pleasure. Choices made by the id alone tend to be child-like and may be irrational.

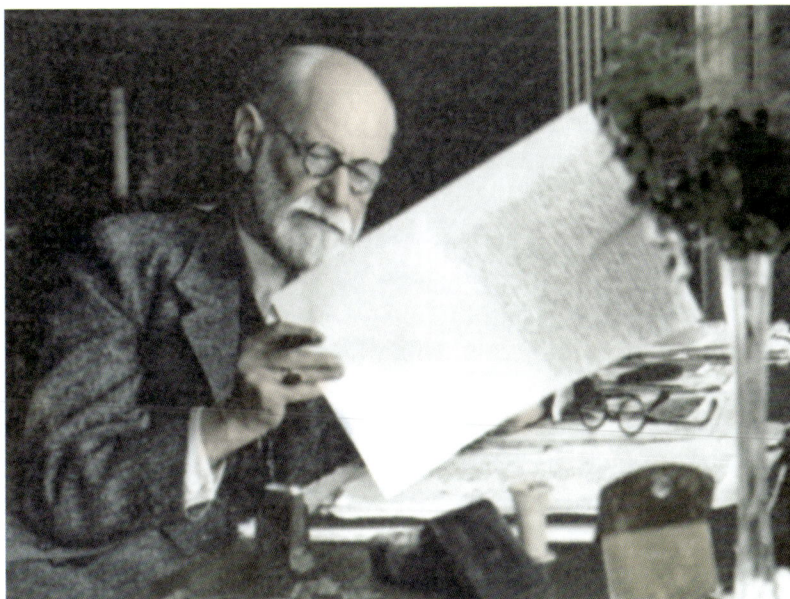

Austrian psychologist Sigmund Freud theorized that the mind contains conscious and unconscious levels; bad memories are repressed and stored unconsciously but may still affect behavior. © PHOTO RESEARCHERS/ALAMY.

The Ego. A primarily conscious part of the psyche, the ego develops during the second half of an infant's first year, and deals with reality. Through planning and decision making, which is also called secondary process thinking, the ego learns that operating on the id level is generally not very effective in the long term. The ego operates through realistic thinking, or on the reality principle. The ego attempts to regulate the id and superego.

The Superego. The superego, which develops throughout childhood, operates more or less as a person's conscience. According to Freud, the superego is the part of the mind that houses the rules and expectations of society, a person's goals, and how the person wants to behave (called the ego-ideal). While the id and ego are considered characteristics of the individual, the superego is based more on outside influences, such as family and society. For example, as children grow up, they will learn which actions and behaviors are not acceptable; from this new knowledge, they learn how to act to win the praise or affection of parents.

Psychoanalytic theory and psychoanalysis are based on Freud's second theory of neurotic anxiety, which is the reaction of the ego when a previously repressed id impulse pushes to express itself. The unconscious part of the ego may encounter a situation that reminds it of a repressed childhood conflict, often related to a sexual or aggressive impulse, and is overcome by overwhelming tension. Psychoanalytic therapy tries to remove the earlier repression and helps the patient resolve the childhood conflict through the use of adult reality.

Free Association. Raising repressed conflicts occurs through different psychoanalytic techniques, one of which is called free association. In free association, the patient reclines on a couch, facing away from the analyst. The analyst sits near the patient's head and often takes notes during a session. The patient is encouraged to talk about whatever comes to mind, without censoring their thoughts. Eventually defenses held by the patient lessen, and a bond of trust between analyst and patient is established.

Dream Analysis. Another technique often used in psychoanalysis is dream analysis because Freud believed that ego defenses are relaxed during sleep, allowing repressed material to enter the sleeper's consciousness. Since these repressed thoughts are so threatening they cannot be experienced in their actual form; the thoughts are disguised in dreams. The dreams, then, become symbolic and significant to the patient's psychoanalytic work.

Transference. Transference is a patient's response to the analyst that is not in keeping with the analyst-patient relationship but seems, instead, to resemble ways of behaving toward significant people in the patient's past. For example, as a result of feeling neglected as children, patients may feel that they must impress the analyst in order to keep the analyst present. Through observation of these transferred attitudes, the analyst gains insight into the childhood origin of repressed conflicts.

One focus of psychoanalysis is the analysis of defenses. The therapist studies the patient's defense mechanisms, which are the ego's unconscious way of warding off a confrontation with anxiety. The analyst points out defensive behavior to stimulate patients to realize that they are avoiding looking at an issue or conflict.

Psychoanalytic sessions between patients and their analysts may occur as frequently as five times a week. This frequency is necessary at the beginning of the relationship in order to establish trust between patient and analyst and achieve a level of comfort that allows repressed conflicts to be uncovered and discussed.

Psychodynamic Therapy

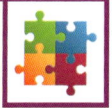

In 1946, psychodynamic therapy was developed in part through the work of Franz Gabriel Alexander, M.D., and Thomas Morton French, M.D., supporters of a briefer analytic therapy than Freud's psychoanalytic theory. Influenced by such Freudian concepts as the defense mechanism and unconscious motivation, psychodynamic therapy is more active than Freudian therapy and focuses more on present problems and relationships than on childhood conflicts. A shorter, less intensive therapy, the session frequency and the patient's body position during therapy matter less than what the patient says and does. With support from the therapist, patients in psychodynamic therapy examine the true sources of their tension and unhappiness by facing repressed feelings and eventually resolving them.

Humanistic and Existential Therapies Humanistic and existential therapies are based on the belief that disordered behavior can be overcome by increasing patients' own awareness of their motivations and needs. Whereas psychoanalysis assumes that human nature (the id) is something in need of restraint, humanistic and existential therapists place more emphasis on a person's freedom of choice. Humanistic and existential therapists believe that free will is a valuable trait and a gift to be used wisely.

Analytical Psychology. Carl Gustav Jung (1887–1961) helped to develop analytical psychology, which is a mixture of Freudian and humanistic psychology. Jung believed that the role of the unconscious was very important in human behavior. In addition to the individual unconscious, Jung said there is a collective unconscious that acts as a storage area for all the experiences that all people have had over the centuries. Jung believed that all people have masculine and feminine traits and he considered spiritual and religious needs as important as physical and sexual needs.

Analytical psychology organizes personality types into groups; the familiar terms "extroverted," or acting out, and "introverted," or turning oneself inward, are Jungian terms used to describe personality traits. Developing a purpose, decision-making, and setting goals are other components of Jung's theory. Whereas Freud believed that a person's current and future behavior is based on experiences of the past, Jungian theorists often focus on dreams, fantasies, and an analysis of unconscious processes so the patient can ultimately integrate them into conscious thought and deal with them. Much of the Jungian technique is based on bringing the unconscious into the conscious.

In explaining personality, Jung said there are three levels of consciousness: the conscious, the personal unconscious, and the collective unconscious.

The conscious is the only level of which a person is directly aware. This awareness begins at birth and continues throughout life. At one point, the conscious experiences a stage called individuation, in which people strive to be different from others and assert themselves as individuals. The goal of individuation is to know oneself wholly and completely. This is accomplished, in part, by bringing unconscious material to the conscious.

The personal unconscious is the landing area of the brain for the thoughts, feelings, experiences, and perceptions that are not picked up by the ego. Repressed personal conflicts or unresolved issues are also stored here. Jung wove this concept into his psychoanalytic theory: often thoughts, memories, and other material in the personal unconscious are associated with each other and form an involuntary theme. Jung assigned the term "complex" to describe this theme.

The idea of the collective unconscious is one that separates Jung's theory of psychotherapy from other theories. Jung said the collective unconscious is made up of images and ideas that are independent of the material in one's personal consciousness. Also present in the collective unconscious are instincts, or strong motivations that are present from birth, and archetypes, which are universally known images or symbols that predispose an individual to have a specific feeling or thought about that image. Archetypes will often show themselves in the form of archetypal images, such as the archetype of death or the archetype of the old woman; death's definition is pretty clear (death equals death) and the archetype of the old woman is often used as a representation of wisdom and age.

Adlerian Psychology. Alfred Adler (1870–1937) became interested in psychology while working as a general medical practitioner. Adler wanted to learn about his patients' social and psychological situations, so he became a psychiatrist (a medical doctor who specializes in the area of the mind). This interest in the whole person was to affect his future work for years to come.

Although at first a member of Freud's psychoanalytic circle, Adler soon branched out on his own and was interested in the study of the subjectivity of perception as well as the importance of social factors as opposed to the importance of biological factors emphasized by Freud. Adler's view of personality stressed the importance of the person as a whole and the individual's interaction with surrounding society. He saw the person as a goal-directed, creative individual responsible for his or her own future.

Because he had been quite ill as a child, Adler had to overcome his own feelings of extreme inferiority (feeling less worthy than others) throughout his childhood. As a result, his theories stressed working toward superiority, but not in an antisocial sense. Instead, he viewed people as tied to their surroundings; Adler claimed that a person's fulfillment was based on doing things for the "social good." Like Jung, Adler also argued the importance of working toward personal goals in therapy.

Adler's work focused on helping patients get over the "illogical expectations" they had for themselves and their lives. He believed that to feel better one must increase one's focus on rational thinking. This belief followed the Jungian theory that the goal of one's life should be individuation, or the conscious realization of one's psychological reality—a reality unlike any other, unique to only that person. As patients become more and more aware of themselves, they combine the unconscious and conscious parts of themselves, thereby becoming stronger and more emotionally whole.

Believing that a person's growth was based on relationships with family during the early years of development, Adler's interest in psychological growth, the prevention of problems, and the improvement of society influenced the creation of child development centers and parent education.

Techniques and Goals of Adlerian Therapy. Crucial to the Adlerian therapy technique is the establishment of a good therapeutic relationship between therapist and patient, one based on respect and mutual trust. In order for this to happen, therapists and patients must share the same goals for their relationships. This often includes encouragement from the therapists that patients can indeed reach their goals by working with their therapists.

Choosing a Therapist

Deciding to begin therapy can be a big enough decision, but choosing a therapist can be just as difficult. Talking to someone one hardly knows, about intensely personal subjects and feelings, is difficult for anyone. Finding the right therapist can take time and patience until one feels the right connection.

Finding a therapist may require a bit of detective work. One's family physician is a good person to ask for the names of prospective therapists. School guidance counselors and clergy members also may be able to make referrals to therapists.

There are options, too, when deciding what kind of therapist to choose. A psychiatrist, along with being a therapist, is also a medical doctor, and can prescribe medication. Clinical psychologists, counselors, pastoral counselors, and social workers also provide therapy, as do marriage and family therapists, art and music therapists, and other kinds of practitioners.

When choosing a therapist it is important to remember that it is fine to be selective; a successful therapeutic relationship requires trust, mutual respect, sensitivity, and understanding.

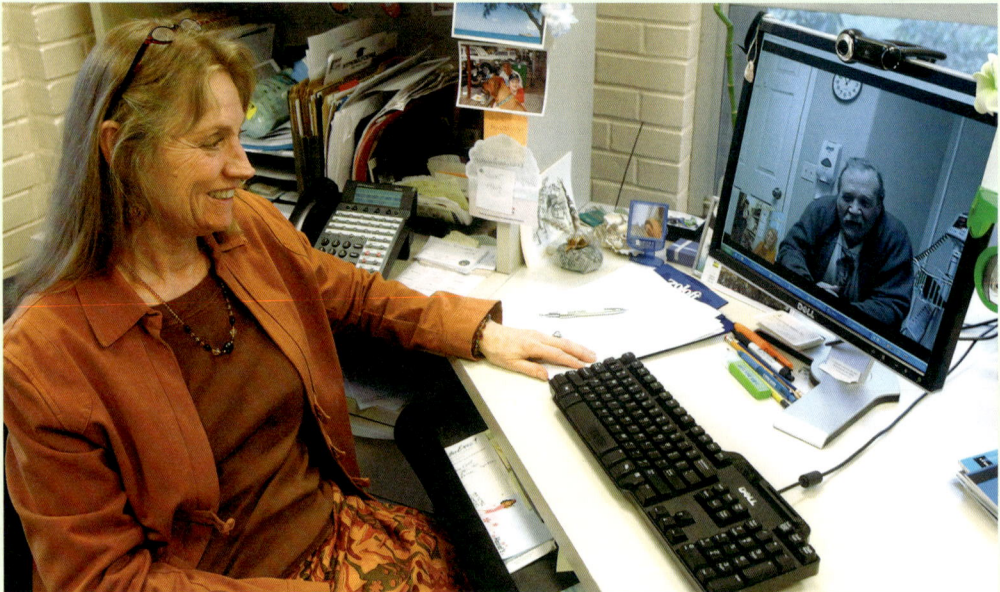

A patient meets with a mental health nurse practitioner via computer teleconference. Though some people may feel more comfortable in the traditional setting of a therapist's office, many patients who are unable to get to an office (or just prefer to use their computer to connect with their therapist) are able to access mental health care online. In addition, some may want to "interview" a therapist online to see if they are compatible with the chosen therapist before committing to seeing them in person. © AP PHOTO/THE NEWS-REVIEW/ROB MCCALLUM.

Therapists may also introduce patients to any signs of self-abusive behaviors, such as resisting or missing therapy sessions. Above all, Adlerian therapists are supportive and empathetic (understanding) to patients; as patients gradually discuss more and more with their therapists, the Adlerians develop knowledge of the lifestyles of their patients. Empathetic responses on the therapists' part often reflect a developed understanding of patients' lifestyles. One of the most important goals of Adlerian therapy is the patient's increase in social interests, as well as an increase in self-awareness and self-confidence.

Existential Therapy Another insight therapy, existential therapy, is based on the philosophical theory of existentialism, which emphasizes the importance of existence, including one's responsibility for one's own psychological existence. One important component of this theory is dealing with life themes instead of techniques; more than other therapies, existential therapy looks at patients' self-awareness and their ability to look beyond the immediate problems and events in their lives and focus instead on problems of human existence.

The concepts of existential therapy were based on the writings of European philosophers, such as Soren Kierkegaard (1813–1855), Friedrich Nietzsche (1844–1900), Karl Jaspers (1883–1969), Martin Heidegger (1889–1976), and Jean-Paul Sartre (1905–1980).

The existential therapist helps patients become more aware of themselves and the results of their actions so that they can take more responsibility for their lives and fulfill their potential.

Person-Centered Therapy Person-centered therapy was developed by American psychologist Carl Rogers. Rogers's therapy is based on four stages: the developmental stage, the nondirective stage, the client-centered stage, and the person-centered stage.

Person-centered therapy looks at assumptions made about human nature and how people can try to understand these assumptions. Like other humanistic therapists, Rogers believed that people should be responsible for themselves, even when they are troubled. Person-centered therapy takes a positive view of patients, believing that they tend to move toward being fully functioning instead of wallowing in their problems.

Techniques and Goals of Person-Centered Therapy. Person-centered therapy is based more on a way of being rather than a therapy technique. Focusing on understanding and caring instead of diagnosis and advice, Rogers believed that change could take place if only a few criteria were met:

1. The patient must be anxious or incongruent (lacking harmony) and be in contact with the therapist.

2. The therapist must be genuine; that is, a therapist's words and feelings must agree.

3. The therapist must accept the patient and care unconditionally for him or her. In addition, the therapist must understand the patient's thoughts and experiences and relay this understanding to the patient.

Rogerian therapists follow the nondirective approach. The therapist cannot provide the answers because the patient must come to conclusions alone. The therapist does not ask questions in a person-centered therapy session, as they may hamper the patient's personal growth, the goal of this therapy.

Gestalt Therapy Gestalt psychology rose from the work of Frederich S. Perls (1893–1970), who felt that a focus on perception and on the development of the whole individual were important. Gestalt therapy has both humanistic and existential aspects; Perls's contemporaries primarily rejected it because Perls disagreed with some of the basic concepts of psychoanalytic theory, such as the importance of the libido and its various transformations in the development of mental disorders. Originally developed in the 1940s, the overall concepts of the Gestalt theory state that people are basically good, and that this goodness should be allowed to show itself; also, psychological problems originate in frustrations and denials of this innate goodness.

Gestalt therapy focuses on the present moment—an awareness of the here and now, and the belief that it is only possible for people to truly know themselves in relation to the world around them. Gestalt therapists feel their approach is uniquely suited to responding to the difficulties and challenges of modern daily life, both in its ability to relieve distress and by helping people realize their full potential.

Techniques and Goals of Gestalt Therapy. Gestalt therapists focus on the creative aspects of people, instead of their problematic parts. There is a focus on the present rather than the past; what is most important for the patient is what is happening in therapy at that time. If the past enters a session and creates problems for the Gestalt patient, it is brought into the present and discussed. Gestalt therapy discourages examination of the past when it is an attempt to escape responsibility for decisions made in the present. The therapist sometimes forces or even bullies patients into an awareness of every detail of the present situation.

Perls created quite a few techniques for patients, but one well-known practice is the empty chair technique, where a patient projects and then faces those projections. For example, a patient may have unresolved feelings about a parent's early death. The patient in Gestalt therapy will sit facing an empty chair and pretend that he is facing the dead parent. The patient can then consciously face, and eventually overcome, unresolved feelings or conflicts toward that parent.

The goal of Gestalt therapy is to help patients understand and accept their needs and fears as well as increase awareness of how they keep themselves from reaching their goals and taking care of their needs. The Gestalt therapist also strives to help patients view the world in a nonjudgmental way. Concentration on the "here and now" and on the patient as responsible for his or her actions and behavior is the desired end result.

Cognitive and Behavior Therapies

Cognition is the term used for the mental processes of perceiving, recognizing, conceiving, judging, and reasoning. Cognitive theory is based on the idea that the learning process is very complex, and one's belief system and ways of thinking are very important when it comes to determining and affecting behavior and feelings.

Psychoanalyst Aaron Beck (1921–) developed cognitive therapy. Beck was intrigued by how people spoke to themselves through their own self-communication system. When his patients experienced thoughts that they were hardly aware of, and these thoughts did not seem to stem from the free association technique practiced in sessions, Beck encouraged patients to focus on these thoughts, which he called automatic thoughts. These unformed thoughts were often connected to unpleasant feelings or memories.

Through the isolation of and focus on these unformed thoughts, Beck was able to identify negative themes that characterized the way patients considered both present and past situations. From these unformed thoughts, patients formed rules for themselves, which Beck called schemas. These schemas, especially within depressed people, were self-defeating and were often negative.

Techniques and Goals of Cognitive Therapy Like Alfred Adler, Aaron Beck used direct dialogue with the patient. Cognitive therapy is based on the idea that negative feelings and activities are caused by irrational beliefs. For example, a child may believe that in order to win the love of his parents he must be a "perfect" son or daughter. This, of course, is an irrational thought—no one can be absolutely perfect.

Through a technique called rational-emotive therapy, cognitive therapists guide their patients to challenge their irrational beliefs and assist them to replace them with new, more positive ones. In the case of the "perfect" son, a cognitive therapist would help him see that although it would be great if he could be perfect, he doesn't have to be without faults to earn the love of his parents.

Cognitive therapists see the patients' past knowledge as "perceptual funnels" through which they view their experiences. Patients are guided to fit new information into an organized network of already accumulated knowledge, called schema. New life information may fit the schema; if not, the patients reorganize the new information to fit the schema. In this way, conflicts and issues are unearthed, discussed, and conquered.

Behavior Therapy American psychologist John B. Watson (1878–1958) felt that psychology was the study of observable behavior instead of an examination of patients' subjective experiences. Behaviorism focuses on the study of this observable behavior instead of on consciousness.

Behavior therapy has its history in the experimental psychology and learning processes of humans and animals. Its main focus is to change certain behaviors instead of uncovering unconscious conflicts or problems. It is based on the theory that abnormal behavior is made up of responses learned the same way that normal behavior is learned. Through behaviorism, therapists use ways of learning new behaviors to help patients.

Operant Conditioning. Operant conditioning focuses on the background and results of behavior. The operant theory, based on the work of E. L. Thorndike (1874–1949) and B. F. Skinner, formed the roots of modern behavior therapy.

Operant conditioning is a type of learning based on the effects of consequences on behavior, where one's behavior is changed by systematically changing the surrounding circumstances. Thorndike developed a principle called the law of effect, which says that behavior

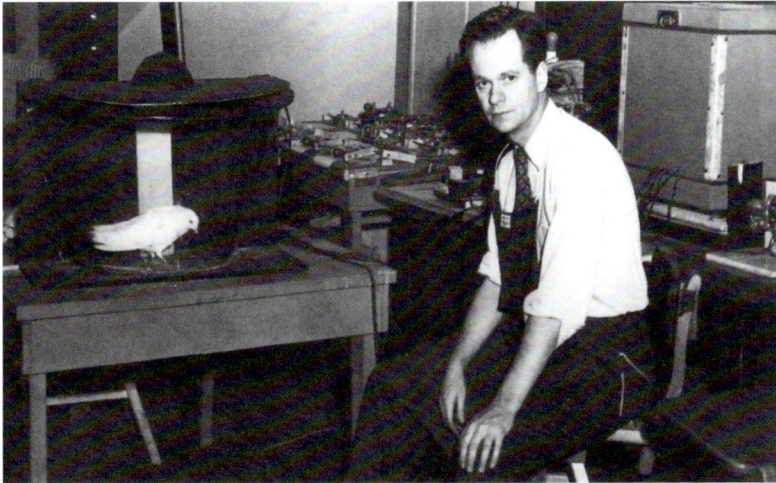

followed by consequences that are satisfying to the subject will be repeated, and that behavior followed by negative consequences will be discouraged.

Skinner introduced the concept of operant conditioning. He adjusted Thorndike's law of effect by shifting the focus from the linking of stimuli and responses to the relationships between those responses and their consequences. He also introduced the concept of a discriminative stimulus, or an external event that tells an animal or human that if a certain behavior is performed, a certain consequence will occur.

A classic example of operant conditioning involves the Skinner box, wherein a subject, often a small animal such as a pigeon, is placed into a closed box with a box of lighted knobs. The psychologist records the number of the subject's pecks at each light. For example, if the pigeon has been deprived of water, it will peck at the knob corresponding to water more times than it pecks at other knobs. The subject can even be trained to peck at specific colored lights by reinforcing one knob over another.

Modeling. Modeling, another behavior therapy tool, is the learning of a behavior by observing and imitating it. This is especially apparent in children, who learn a significant amount through modeling. Modeling is also a very effective treatment for severely disturbed patients because it teaches them new social behavior that can improve their functioning in the world.

Healthy Living, 2nd Edition

Modeling uses cognitive behaviors (perception, reasoning, etc.) to effectively absorb the modeled behavior. Modeling has developed and has been effectively used as a form of cognitive-behavioral therapy because it provides the subject with a "code" or plan in which to learn the new behavior. Researchers have learned that when subjects have a model or plan to follow, the new information is better retained. Also, the use of this code or plan helps subjects pattern their own actions on what they have seen modeled.

Cognitive-Behavioral Therapy Cognitive-behavioral therapy (CBT) is based on the idea that thinking influences emotions and behavior—that feelings and actions begin with thoughts. So if patients have unwanted feelings and behaviors then it is important for them to identify the thinking that is causing the feelings and behaviors and to learn how to replace their thinking with thoughts that produce better reactions. CBT is based on the idea that it is possible to change the way people feel and act even if their circumstances do not change. It teaches the advantages of feeling, at worst, calm when faced with undesirable situations. Patients learn that they will face undesirable events and circumstances whether they become troubled about the events or not. When they are troubled about events or circumstances, they have two problems—the troubling event or circumstance and the troubling feelings about the event or circumstance. Patients learn that when they do not become troubled about trying events and circumstances they can reduce the number of problems they face by half.

CBT is a short-term therapy with patients receiving an average of just 16 sessions. Compared to other forms of therapy, CB therapists tend to offer more instruction than other therapists and usually assign "homework," in the form of reading assignments and practicing the techniques learned.

Rational-Emotive Behavior Therapy Albert Ellis (1913–2007) believed that antisocial, negative feelings and activity are caused by irrational beliefs based on a code one makes for oneself about how to live. People mistakenly put extreme demands on themselves and those around them, as when a person who strives to be perfect makes a mistake and feels overwhelmingly terrible; the person will use that internal communication system to punish himself. In addition, people will occasionally attempt to make sense of what occurs around them, and these discoveries may cause conflict. Ellis stressed the importance of the therapist's attention to the patient's beliefs instead of the cause of the conflict.

Rational-emotive behavior therapists differ in the ways they use to persuade patients to adopt new ways of communicating with themselves. Some therapists have been known to tease, coerce, or bully their patients into realizing new forms of self-communication. Others suggest that patients discuss their irrational beliefs and then gently guide them toward a more rational way of living. With this behavior therapy technique, Ellis and his supporters helped their patients rethink their original, negative beliefs and guided them to restructure those thoughts or beliefs. For example, the patient who made the mistake is coached into rethinking the scenario and inserts a realistic thought: although it would be nice to be perfect, everybody makes mistakes at some point.

Behavioral Medicine Behavioral medicine is the study of ideas and knowledge taken from medicine and behavioral science (psychology). It incorporates the knowledge of many different practitioners, from social workers to psychiatrists and researchers. It is used to understand physical and mental illness as well as to prevent and treat psychophysiological disorders (physical maladies caused by emotional distress, such as stress and other illnesses that involve the psyche). Behavioral medicine has also been used to study and treat acute and chronic pain.

Biofeedback. Biofeedback uses sensitive machines to provide patients with information about their blood pressure, skin temperature, brain waves, and other bodily functions. The patient, painlessly hooked up to these machines, is given an auditory or visual sign when there is a change in his or her condition. Learning the signal before blood pressure rises, for example, can help patients train themselves to identify the behaviors or situations that might be causing blood pressure to rise.

Biofeedback can be a very effective way to combat stress-induced conditions, such as anxiety, hives, and tension headaches, but it has also proven helpful for patients with attention-deficit disorder (ADD), depression, and other emotional disturbances.

Pain Management. Adapting to pain does not seem like something one would want to learn at all, but for many people pain is a part of every day. Dealing with that maladaptive pain (pain that seriously limits one's enjoyment of life) without it taking over can be difficult. Researchers have learned that if patients are distracted from their pain, the pain

Reality Therapy

Based on the control theory, which states that people are responsible for their lives and actions, reality therapy was established to help people make choices, both simple and difficult, and ultimately control their behavior.

Psychiatrist William Glasser (1925–) developed this form of therapy because he was dissatisfied with psychoanalysis' belief that patients should deny responsibility for their behavior and instead blame others and their past for their problems. Glasser stresses that relationships between therapists and patients should be friendly, open, and accepting. As patients commit to therapy, Glasser believes they can be guided toward altering their ways of thinking and feeling.

In reality therapy, talking about one's feelings is accepted, but is not a major focus of the therapy. Instead, Glasser focuses on helping people make changes in their lives and maintaining those changes. The therapist, according to Glasser, should not accept excuses from patients, as this would hinder the healing process.

This therapy technique has attracted the attention of therapists, school counselors, substance abuse counselors, and corrections employees. Institutional populations such as mental hospitals and prisons, with their more challenging populations, have also had success with the use of reality therapy.

Reality therapy has specific goals. It aims to help patients find feelings of belonging, freedom, power, and fun. The therapist meets with patients to assess whether their needs are being met and works with them to attain these feelings and experiences, reestablishing or perhaps even establishing for the first time positive life experiences.

may be lessened when it occurs or may not even be felt at all. Cognitive psychologists have also found that, since everyone has a limited amount of attention to channel toward one stimulus, distracting patients from the pain and toward something else guides them to focusing all attention on the other stimulus. This human limitation can actually prove beneficial to the pain sufferers.

Pharmacotherapy

Pharmacotherapy, or drug therapy, is often used to treat people with mental illness. Whether to treat anxiety or depression or another more serious condition such as schizophrenia, there seems to be a pill for every affliction. Conducted under a doctor's supervision, drug therapy may be a very effective way of combating some types of mental illness. Often, medication is used in conjunction with regular therapy sessions.

Generally patients remain on the prescription drug treatment until there is a marked improvement or decline in the patient's condition over a period of time, usually a few months. Then there may be a change in medication (if a decline in mental health is experienced) or a decrease in dose to test whether the patient's mental stability remains or fluctuates. A positive mood change can mean either the beginning of the end of the patient's drug therapy or the need for a change. Sometimes it takes a few tries with different medications until the right one is found. Sometimes the medication works for a while, but then becomes ineffective. Sometimes it's a matter of adjusting the patient's dose or adding a supplementary medication to the therapy plan.

In recent years, some researchers have questioned whether some drugs, such as antidepressants, are overprescribed. An analysis of six studies covering 30 years of antidepressant drug treatment suggests that people with severe depression benefit most from antidepressant medications, while there is little or no benefit for people with the less-severe symptoms of mild depression. The study found that the benefit of antidepressant medication was no better than placebo (a pill that contains no active ingredients) for people with mild to moderate depression.

Nontraditional Mental Health Therapy Techniques

Nontraditional or alternative medicine also offers a variety of therapies that may effectively treat different kinds of mental illness and their symptoms.

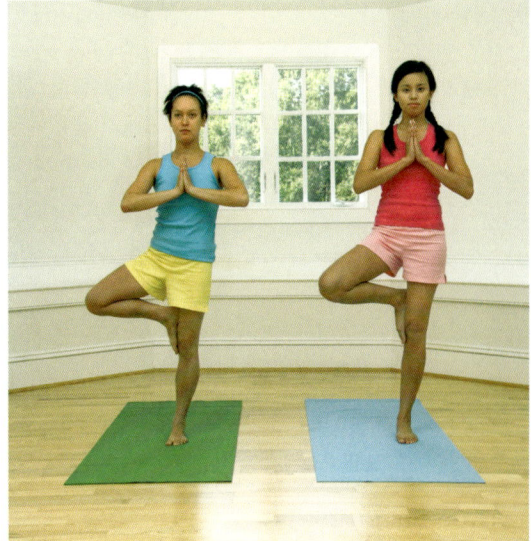

Two young women maintain balance while doing yoga tree pose. © IOPHOTO/ SHUTTERSTOCK.COM.

Yoga First practiced in India thousands of years ago, yoga has grown in popularity in the United States. There are different kinds of yoga including Hatha yoga, Iyengar yoga, Sahaja yoga, and Kundalini yoga.

Although often seen as a form of exercise, yoga is also used in many cultures as a way of maintaining physical as well as mental health. The benefits of yoga are found in the asanas, or poses, and in pranayama, or the breathing exercises. Performed properly and practiced regularly, they can bring positive changes in the body. Although they may look easy, asanas are a challenge: in a subtle relationship between body and mind, they engage several muscle groups at once and require a huge amount of concentration, focus, and strength.

There are obvious physical benefits to practicing yoga, such as an increase in muscle tone, strength, and flexibility, but this centuries-old practice also regulates and brings oxygen to all areas of the body. If there are problems in certain parts of the body, specific poses can be done to expedite the healing process in that area.

The breathing-exercise, meditative (pranayama) stage of the class may precede or follow the asanas. Sometimes a meditation or relaxation-like phase will occur both at the beginning and at the end of the class.

Yoga's main goal is to attain harmony and peace between the body, mind, and spirit; yoga means "union" in the ancient language of Sanskrit, and each

All forms of therapy can produce positive results. Therapy alone, drug treatment, or a combination of the two can help most people feel better. Patience, an open mind, and a strong therapist-patient relationship based on trust and respect are all important, however, the key to success is to find a form of treatment that works and to keep at it.

pose is created to harmonize specific body systems and parts with the mind and spirit. One pose, for example, may have the benefits of strengthening the back muscles, but, if done properly, may also release repressed fear held in the body. Another pose urges along the cleaning process of the liver while it also lengthens the spine and carries fresh blood to the liver and brain.

How, then, does yoga work as a form of therapy? As yoga students practice yoga, incorporating both the asanas and the meditation or breathing exercises, they realize, over a few weeks, a decrease in anxiety levels, and a calming, "at peace" feeling. Studies have shown that people with anxiety disorders, depression, and even psychosis have experienced an improvement in their mental health from practicing yoga. Of course, an improvement in one's physical appearance from the practice of yoga can boost one's self-confidence, but yoga can also bring a healthy feeling of order to the inside of the body as well.

Meditation Contrary to popular belief, meditation is much more than just sitting quietly. In fact, learning how to meditate is hard work, but the benefits of meditation can have lasting effects. This age-old practice has even found popularity among people looking for help with mental health problems.

Therapists report that people who meditate experience decreases in anxiety and stress levels, addictive behaviors, and depressions. Sometimes meditation is practiced along with other nontraditional therapy techniques, such as yoga. However it is practiced, the most important aspect of meditation is concentration.

To attain the intense concentration needed for effective meditation, patients often choose an object, word, or phrase on which to focus and center their attention. Some kinds of meditation incorporate props, such as lit candles, for focusing. Others suggest repeating a word or phrase over and over, such as "ohm," which is used in Hindu traditions. Any word, though, will do; some people will repeat the word "love" or "peace." Once concentration is attained, the next step—unbroken attention (meditation)— should follow. (It is important to note here that getting to this point is a challenge. With meditation, patience is a virtue. Also, if people find their thoughts wandering from the chosen focus, which is normal, they should allow the uninterrupted thoughts to enter and then leave the mind, followed by a gentle self-guide back to the original word, phrase, or object.) Once this state of meditation is reached, a higher state of consciousness, sometimes called contemplation, is the next level. This may not be necessary for the beginner; benefits will still be felt even if this higher consciousness is not immediately achieved.

Meditation can be a great way to increase focus and reduce anxiety and other mood disorders such as depression. Meditation is not something that can be practiced once with expected results; like yoga and other non-traditional medical techniques, it requires focus, patience, and dedication.

Bioenergetics (Body/Mind Therapy) Bioenergetics, also called body/mind therapy, is a body-related psychotherapy developed by American doctor Alexander Lowen (1910–2008). Lowen was a student of Wilhelm Reich (1897–1957), a famous Austrian psychotherapist.

Influenced by Reich's theories, Lowen argued that the body, mind, and spirit are all interdependent and reflective. By practicing special exercises and verbal therapy, the body and mind can be freed from negative actions, called restrictive holding patterns. Bioenergetic therapists try to help their patients reach this freedom of body and mind.

Bioenergetics is based on the belief that personality is made of biological urges and conscious thought, or will. Lowen believed that emotional problems develop when biological impulses are not consciously expressed because of fear. Bioenergetic exercises aim to loosen rigid muscles and break down defenses so that the true self can emerge. These exercises also increases the amount of psychophysical energy (energy from the body and the mind); Lowen calls this bioenergy.

Breaking down this defense occurs gradually and, as the body feels more alive, repressed feelings are released. The verbal (talk) therapy aspect of the technique happens throughout the defense-lifting process, allowing the person to combine new thoughts and physical feelings into his or her life.

Bioenergetics begins with the therapist and patient having a conversation, but then moves directly into the exercises, or bodywork. Patients wear close-fitting clothing so the therapist can see how the body changes as it moves. The exercises include lying, sitting, and standing in ways that increase the areas of stress in the body. Deep breathing during the session is encouraged because it pulls a large amount of bioenergy into the body, releasing repressed emotions. This energy is compared to an electric current, and can actually be seen by both therapist and patient as vibrations in muscles.

Throughout the exercises, the bioenergetic therapist might touch or massage certain areas of the patient's body that seem to resist release. At certain points during the session, the patient is also reminded to make sounds (as part of the verbal therapy); the release of sounds sends more bioenergy through the body.

Since the release of defenses in the body happens over a period of time and not all at once, bioenergetics is a long-term therapy, but it helps many people to control or combat feelings of anxiety, depression, or other kinds of emotional upset.

Creative Arts Therapies Unlike talk therapies, art therapy relies on the use of making art and art interpretation rather than solely on verbal communication to uncover and explore feelings, emotions, and ideas. Art therapies use some form of creative expression to promote change in people's mental health. Some of these therapies include art, drama, dance, poetry, and music. This form of therapy aims to promote an increase in self-esteem, self-expression, and improved social interactions.

With its roots in psychotherapy, art therapy first became a tool for releasing hidden emotions in the unconscious through spontaneous art. It proved especially useful with people unable, unwilling, or unlikely to express their feelings in conventional, problem-oriented, and solution-focused psychotherapy. Art therapy became widely used, with great success, by mental health practitioners working with children and persons who had suffered physical or sexual abuse. More recently, interest in the connection of mind, body, and spirit has lead to explorations through the art process of emotional conflicts, physical symptoms, and personal growth.

Early art therapists made meaning of the patient's art, and developed strategies to help people uncover and face the cause of their symptoms. Over time, the focus of art therapy shifted. There was greater recognition of the value and importance of the patient taking personal responsibility for analysis and change. The freer, open-ended, and more fluid approach to art therapy appeared better suited for uncovering and communicating possibilities and opportunities for change. Furthermore, modern art therapy enabled patients and therapists to benefit from the process of art making as well as their efforts to interpret the art work.

Art Therapy. Art therapy is used to help patients overcome emotional conflicts and become more self-aware. The art therapist guides patients as they use art materials, such as pastels or crayons, to express themselves, but clay, paper, or finger paints may also be used, depending on the issue being addressed. These specially selected materials can be used to express what is in patients' minds before they are able to put it into words.

Art therapy can provide a positive feeling of expression within patients as well as allow a physical release of creative energy as work is being created. If a specific topic is not immediately apparent, the therapist might suggest a topic for expression, such as the patient's family or a vivid childhood memory.

Dance and Movement Therapy. Using the freedom of movement, dance therapy can help patients express themselves through virtually any form of movement, no matter how spontaneous. Therapists' approaches to patients are creative, but must also result from observation of patients' immediate needs through signs like physical tension. The dance or art therapist may also copy patients' actions to relay understanding of certain situations. During dance or movement therapies patients may be asked to respond verbally or to keep moving. The use of rhythm and energy also may help patients who need to release both physical and emotional tension.

Dance therapy has shown success with everyone from professional dancers to autistic children. It allows patients to feel emotional and physiological feelings at the same time and to convey them in a secure, constructive setting.

Music Therapy. Music has been part of human culture more or less since the beginning of time. It has also been associated in the past as having power; in ancient Greece, for example, it was thought to have a special force over one's physical and emotional self. In addition, music has also played a significant role in cultural and religious services. It makes sense, then, that music could be used in therapy.

Today, the calming effect of music is still a by-product of music therapy. Music therapists use the power of music to identify and deal with a wide range of emotional disturbances—everything from drug abuse to schizophrenia and Alzheimer disease.

There is a wide variety of music therapy approaches. Most music therapists have instruments available for patients to use during sessions in their quest for self-expression. Using these instruments, therapists lead exercises to aid the process of uncovering conflict. Often, patients are encouraged to act out spontaneous expressions, even if they might interfere with an exercise. The instruments also may be used as props to describe and act out certain situations. In a classic example, patients might be asked to choose and then manipulate instruments that remind them of family members or difficult situations or feelings.

Psychodrama. Psychodrama, another creative arts therapy technique, has shown to be a very effective therapy form used with other forms of psychotherapy and in crisis intervention.

In psychodrama, the therapist and patient approach a problem as if they were director and playwright, which allows the patient more opportunities to engage with the issue and resolve the conflict. By acting out their problems, patients also experience a deeper level of awareness.

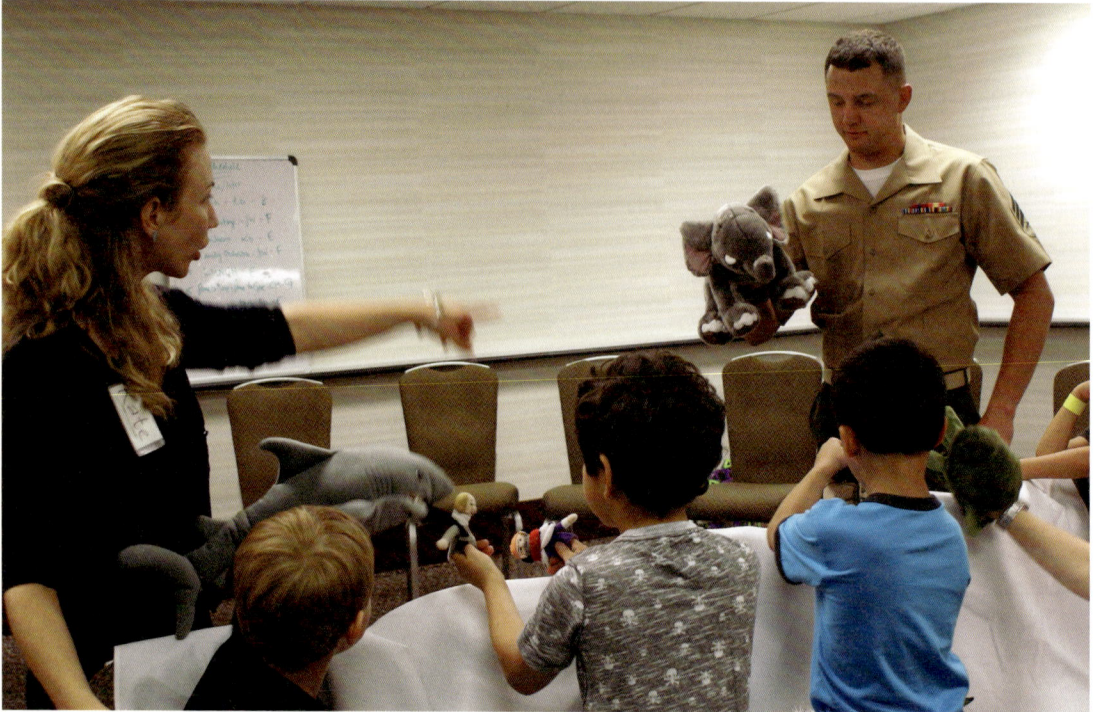

Therapist Kate Dillingham, left, talks with children as Duane Stuckman, a Marine based at the Great Lakes Naval Station, uses a puppet during a role-playing exercise in Chicago. The exercise is part of Operation Oak Tree, a program that offers arts-focused therapy to help military families deal with the emotional stages of deployment. Launched in 2009, the program encourages kids to express their feelings about having mom, dad, or other family deploy. © AP IMAGES/BARBARA RODRIGUEZ.

Developed in the 1930s by Viennese psychiatrist J. L. Moreno (1889–1974), psychodrama has been found to help people suffering from post-traumatic stress disorder, substance abuse, and other conditions requiring long-term hospitalization. The materials used range from classic forms of playwriting, such as Shakespeare, to simpler forms of theater, such as puppet shows. In psychodrama sessions, the therapist keeps close tabs on patients and establishes just the right relationships with them. A patient, for example, might act out a submissive character, such as a mouse, whereas the therapist chooses to be a dominant animal, such as a cat, and acts out that character while observing the patient's reactions. The drama therapist works hard in sessions and goes beyond classic role-playing techniques to work as actor and director.

The goal of psychodrama is for the patient, through acting, to enact life conflicts and derive self-awareness and insight. Other benefits of psychodrama include an increase in creativity, improved interpersonal skills, and an increased ability to solve and resolve problems.

Hypnotherapy Hypnosis is a trancelike state of altered consciousness that resembles sleep but is induced by a person whose suggestions are readily accepted by the subject. In a therapeutic setting, hypnosis is often accompanied by physical relaxation, which can be very helpful when uncovering topics and feelings that produce stress.

There are two approaches to hypnotherapy: the permissive and the indirect. Using the permissive technique, the hypnotherapist treats patients as equals, gently instructing them that they may move along with the hypnosis process if desired (for example, "You may take a deep breath now, if you wish"). The hypnotherapist using the indirect approach, however, would say, "Take a deep breath now." The indirect technique is different from the permissive one in another way: it does not use a formal hypnosis procedure, and the patient is usually unaware that the procedure is happening.

After the initial interview between therapist and patient and an explanation of the realities of hypnosis (for example, that the therapist does not have complete control over the patient's brain, as the media often portrays), the therapist will induce the hypnotic state. This is done through visual imagery; the patient pictures a relaxing situation and is instructed to relive that situation and feeling as much as possible. When the patient reaches some level of trance (often reached while listening to the therapist verbalize the visualization techniques), depending on the level of hypnosis, the patient may be able to recall certain repressed memories.

The use and value of memories recovered by hypnosis remains controversial. In recent years the media have described the disagreements surrounding the existence, nature, and accuracy of recovered memories of child abuse and the responsibility of psychotherapists who may unintentionally create false memories of such abuse.

Although not a form of psychotherapy itself, hypnotherapy has been used successfully to anxiety disorders, mild depression, substance abuse, and sleep disorders.

Therapy Formats

There are a few basic types of therapy, and their characteristics are described below.

Individual Therapy Often the first form of counseling encountered by first-time therapy seekers, individual therapy involves sessions with a therapist and patient. The sessions are usually held regularly and, depending on the kind of therapy chosen, sessions may occur anywhere from one to four times a week. Details of individual therapy sessions (that is, the positions of the patient and therapist in the room, the duration of a session, the nature of the therapist-patient relationship, etc.) vary across different therapy types.

Many patients prefer individual therapy to other forms of therapy because of the one-on-one attention received from the therapist. For others, it may be hard enough for them to express themselves with their therapist, and in a group setting the patient may feel very uncomfortable and not at all like talking.

Individual therapy is often suggested for first-time patients to fully introduce the therapy experience in a gentle, personal manner. Patients may then move on to other forms of therapy or even add a second therapy form to their initial treatment plans.

Marriage and Family Therapy Couples or marriage therapy is often paired with family therapy because of the similar topics discussed in both forms. Today, the term "couples" is used more often than "marital," however, to include the growing number of people who live together in a committed relationship but are not yet married or choose not to marry. Couples therapy and family therapy will be discussed together here because of their similarities.

In both couples and family therapy, the relationship between therapist and patient is not as important as the relationship and interaction between the couple or family members. The goal is to allow the patient to see the partner or family member as he or she really is and not as a product of the patient's repressed emotions about that person. Usually, a conflict between a couple or between family members is a sign of an emotional difficulty in one member of the couple or family; the therapist works to figure out what that conflict might be. Sex therapy, too, is often part of couples therapy, as sexual problems between partners are a common problem; when other conflicts arise within the relationship, a couple's sex life will likely be affected.

In couples and family sessions, patients are encouraged to listen to one another with empathy and to be clear in relaying what they think is being said by the other patient(s) and how they feel about the issues discussed. The therapist's awareness of which stage each patient is in at a certain point of the relationship (at the beginning of a conflict or at a point where a partner or family member is considering leaving the relationship), is also important in planning the therapy strategy.

Many therapists also offer premarital counseling for couples before they get married to help them identify and anticipate potential problems and sources of stress in their relationships. Postmarital therapy, in which separating or divorcing couples seek help in working out their differences can help to minimize stress during negotiation of emotionally-charged issues such as child custody.

Family therapy involves all the members of a nuclear or extended family and may be conducted by a single mental health practitioner, pair, or team of therapists. Co-therapists or teams often include male and female therapists to address gender-related issues or serve as role models through their interactions with one another during sessions for family members. The therapists analyze family interactions and communication and while they do not focus on or side with individual family members they try to enhance awareness and understanding of troubling patterns.

Today family therapy is used to treat a variety of problems such as eating disorders, substance abuse, and adjustment problems stemming from new jobs, schools, or geographic relocation. It is short-term therapy, intended to help families effectively overcome challenges. Example of these include:

- Multigenerational families—problems arising from parents sharing housing with grandparents or homes in which children are reared by grandparents
- Families that face unusual challenges—blended families involving children from multiple marriages, gay couples, and racially mixed families may not experience inter-familial problems but

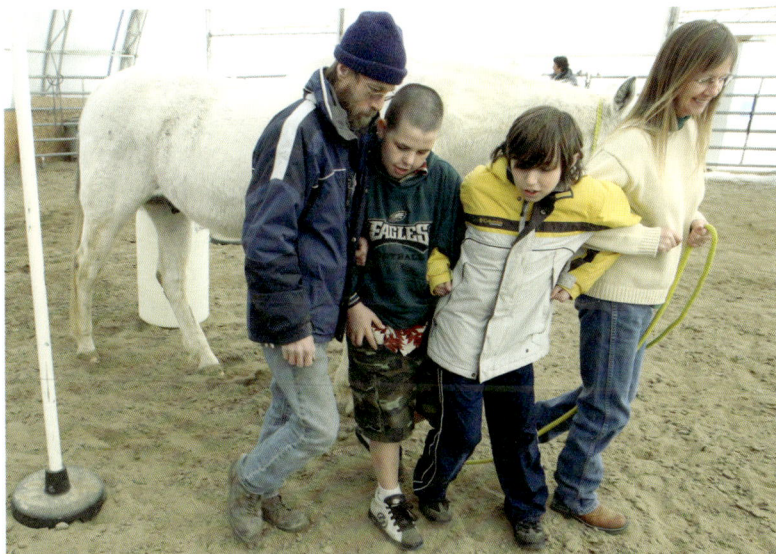

The Herman family, from left, Bob, Jarred, Kaleb, and Kristin, use a combination of family and animal-assisted therapy during an equine (horse) therapy session. The family works together to saddle a horse using only one hand from each parent and getting directions from the two sons. Jarred, who lives in a group home, has completed over 20 equine assistance psychotherapy sessions with his family after traditional therapy failed to address his anger and aggression.
© AP IMAGES/BILLINGS GAZETTE/ PAUL RUHTER.

may require support and assistance to cope with unfavorable or judgmental attitudes expressed by others

- Families that are not supportive of a member suffering from a mental disorder or those that actively undermine the treatment of a family member in individual therapy
- Families in which the identified patient's problems seem to be caused by, or associated with, other family members' problems. The "identified patient" is the family member with the problem that caused the family to enter treatment

While some of family therapy is based on cognitive–behavioral or psychodynamic principles, the most common approach relies on family systems theory. This theory considers the family as the unit of treatment, and focuses on relationships and communication patterns within the family rather than the personality traits or symptoms displayed by individual family members. Family systems theory considers the family as an entity that is more than the sum of its individual members and uses "systems theory" to determine family members' roles within the system as a whole. Problems are addressed by changing or adjusting the system rather than trying to change an individual family member.

One important premise of family systems theory is the idea that families work to maintain their traditional organization and functioning and resist change. Family systems theory suggests that triangular emotional relationships in families serve to maintain homeostasis. When any two family members have problems with one another, they draw in a third member to stabilize their own relationship. Another key concept is the ability of each family member to maintain a sense of self, while remaining emotionally connected to the family. Family systems theory states that healthy families allow and even encourage members to separate and become independent while troubled families may try to prevent individuals from doing that or try to punish those who attempt it.

The aims of family systems therapy include improved insight and communication, awareness and change of troubled behavior patterns, and successful resolution of the problems that prompted the family to enter treatment. The changing definitions and composition of American families have contributed to the increasing popularity of this type of therapy.

Group Therapy Group therapy gathers a small number of people—usually 6–12—to meet regularly to talk, interact, and discuss problems with one another and the therapist who serves as facilitator and group leader.

In some groups two therapists guide group members' processes of self-discovery. Group therapy offers a safe, comfortable setting where members may identify and address problems and emotional issues. It is different from individual therapy because it offers members the chance to counsel and support others. For many people, group therapy is just as effective as individual therapy.

Group therapy provides social acceptance and powerful reassurance that members are not alone—others face similar challenges—and may effectively reduce feelings of being alone. It also provides opportunities to display empathy, practice communication, and other relationship skills in a supportive environment, under the watchful eye of a mental health professional. Finally, through the act of helping group members identify, address, and resolve their problems, group therapy members may gain more self-esteem.

Before entering group therapy, interested patients meet with the group leader or therapist so the therapist can get to know them and the patients can get a feel for what the group sessions will be like. Groups usually meet once a week for one to two hours.

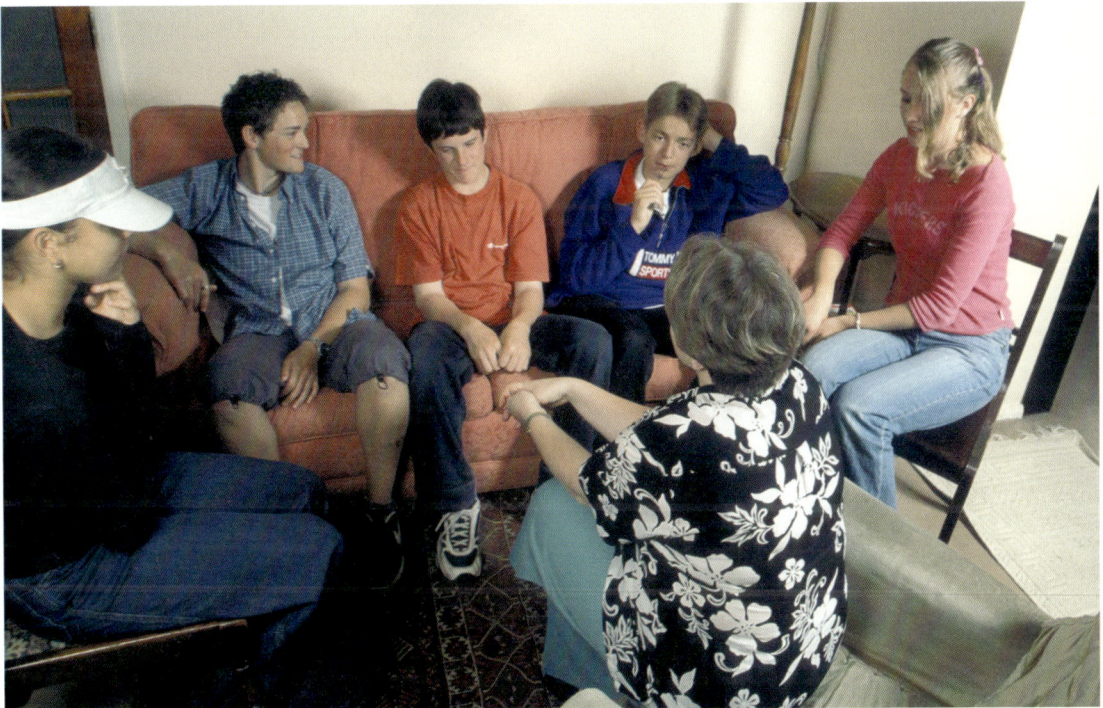

Teens attend a group therapy session with a counselor. © ANGELA HAMPTON PICTURE LIBRARY/ALAMY.

Healthy Living, 2nd Edition

Coping with Death

At one time or another, everyone will experience the death of someone close. The death of a family member or friend and the feelings of shock, loss, anger, depression, and fear may be the most painful and difficult experiences the some people must face. Grief is the term used to describe the many feelings associated with the death of a loved one.

The grieving process is different for everyone. Some people react to the death of a loved one with shock, and seem to be numb. This is an especially common reaction to a sudden or unexpected death such as the loss of a young person as a result of an automobile accident. Sometimes, family members feel angry the person who died. Other times they simply feel pain and emptiness—a great gaping hole left by the death of their loved one. Nearly everyone suffers from sadness or depression.

Funerals, memorial services, and other rites and rituals help families cope with the death of their loved ones. They provide comforting rituals and bring together extended family, friends, and other members of the community to support the grieving family. Although it is never easy to deal with the loss of a family member, it can be less painful if people focus on remembering the good qualities of the person who died; allow themselves to feel hurt and loss, rather than trying to hide from or run away from these feelings; and share their memories and feelings with others.

Much as we might like family members and friends to recover quickly and return to the way they were before the death occurred, allowing them the time to feel the hurt and loss and to fully grieve is very important and necessary for healing. Over time, the terrible pain of the loss will lessen, and those affected will be able to move ahead with their lives. The person who died will not be forgotten but their families and friends will find ways to accept the death of their loved one.

Support groups for adults who have lost a spouse, children who have lost parents, parents who have lost children, and teens who have lost friends can help people share their pain with others who understand their loss and also are grieving. Support groups also offer people the comfort of knowing that they are not alone and that others have some of the same feelings and experiences as they heal from the loss of a loved one.

Once in the group meeting, the hour begins either with one person opening the conversation or with an opening from the therapist. Much less involved than in other therapy forms, the group therapist acts more as mediator, referee, and time clock than anything else. What is important is to get group members to interact among themselves in a constructive manner. Sometimes all members of the group participate, sometimes not, depending on the topic or group members' attitudes that session.

Short-term groups are time limited with a predetermined number of meetings. While long-term or continuing groups may gain and lose members, most short-term groups have a fixed membership throughout their duration. Therapeutic groups operate based on rules governing confidentiality—members may not share the details of therapy sessions with anyone outside of the group. They may also be asked to agree not to socialize with other group members outside of therapy because it might have a harmful effect on the dynamics of the group.

Support Groups Created to educate and protect its members, a support group exists as a way to help people with the same or similar problems and conditions in a group setting. Examples include groups for teenagers, women with breast cancer, and bereavement groups for persons recovering from the loss of a loved one. Some groups are composed of individuals with varying concerns and circumstances. The therapeutic philosophy used in group therapy depends on the group and the training of the therapist. Most groups use psychodynamic, cognitive-behavioral, or Gestalt therapy techniques.

Alcoholics Anonymous (AA). Based partly on the studies of cognitive therapists and techniques of rational-emotive behavior therapy (REBT), Alcoholics Anonymous (AA) has provided help to millions of people who suffer from alcoholism. AA is based on a 12-step program for restructuring one's life as an addict; in these 12 steps addicts admit to, come to terms with, and hopefully conquer their addictions. AA also acts as a support network for alcoholics and recovering alcoholics in the effort to become, and stay, clean and sober.

AA and the 12-step program paved the way for numerous substance-abuse or other kinds of support groups, such as Narcotics Anonymous, Gamblers Anonymous, Overeaters Anonymous, and Bulimics Anonymous. Offshoot support groups, such as Al-Anon, for alcoholics' loved ones, have also developed for the families, partners, and friends of addicts.

Both the support and offshoot support groups can be very helpful for those battling addictive behaviors, whether it is the addicts or their families and friends. As with so many other therapy forms and techniques, benefitting from a support group requires dedication, time, and patience.

Self-Help

Battling and living with a mental illness or other emotional upset can be overwhelming and sometimes very painful. Even with therapy, people may still feel alone and as though their emotions are out of control. Adopting a healthy lifestyle can help to soften the edges of the daily struggle.

- Exercise: Regular exercise can greatly improve symptoms of an emotional disturbance. Not only does it promote good overall health and increase self-esteem and appearance, but it also has been shown to decrease levels of anxiety and depression.

- Sleep: Adequate sleep is crucial when living with a mental illness. During sleep the body has the chance to rebuild, replenish, and rest, which is vital for a healthy body and mind.

- Eat properly: This can be tough; today's busy schedules make it difficult to get enough fruit, vegetables, whole grains, and lean protein each day. But just as sleep is essential to maintaining the body, a healthful diet can provide the brainpower and physical energy needed to live life fully.

- Follow a mental health plan: Whether one lives with an anxiety disorder or full-blown clinical depression, it is important to follow the mental health treatment plan arranged between patient and therapist.

For More Information

BOOKS

Barondes, Samuel. *Making Sense of People: Decoding the Mysteries of Personality.* Upper Saddle River, NJ: FT Press, 2012.

Capacchione, Lucia. *The Art of Emotional Healing.* Boston: Shambhala, 2006.

Capacchione, Lucia. *The Creative Journal for Teens: Making Friends with Yourself,* 2nd ed. Franklin Lakes, NJ: New Page Books, 2002.

Carlseon, Dale. *The Teen Brain Book: Who and What Are You?* Madison, CT: Bick Publishing House, 2004.

Ciarrochi, Joseph, Louise Hayes, and Ann Bailey. *Get Out of Your Mind and Into Your Life for Teens: A Guide to Living an Extraordinary Life.* Oakland, CA: Instant Help, 2012.

Kellerman, Henry. *Personality: How It Forms.* New York: American Mental Health Foundation Books, 2012.

Nettle, Daniel. *Personality: What Makes You the Way You Are.* New York: Oxford University Press, USA, 2009.

Wood, Jeffrey C. *Getting Help: The Complete & Authoritative Guide to Self-Assessment And Treatment of Mental Health Problems.* Oakland, CA: New Harbinger Publications, 2007.

WEB SITES

American Academy of Child and Adolescent Psychiatry. http://www.aacap.org (accessed December 11, 2012).

American Psychiatric Association. http://www.psych.org (accessed December 11, 2012).

National Alliance on Mental Illness. http://www.nami.org (accessed December 11, 2012).

National Mental Health Association. http://www.nmha.org (accessed December 11, 2012).

The Nemours Foundation. "Teens Health: Mind." *KidsHealth.org.* http://www.teenmentalhealth.org/ (accessed December 7, 2012).

"The Teen Brain: Still Under Construction." *National Institute of Mental Health.* http://www.nimh.nih.gov/health/publications/the-teen-brain-still-under-construction/teens-and-the-brain-more-questions-for-research.shtml (accessed December 11, 2012).

Teen Mental Health. http://www.teenmentalhealth.org/ (accessed December 7, 2012).

"Teen Mental Health." *Medline Plus.* http://www.nlm.nih.gov/medlineplus/teenmentalhealth.html (accessed December 7, 2012).

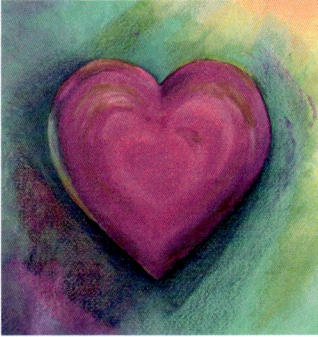

Mental Illness

Introduction **485**

Childhood Disorders **487**

Mood Disorders **503**

Psychotic Disorders **508**

Anxiety Disorders **511**

Other Types of Mental Disorders **521**

For More Information **526**

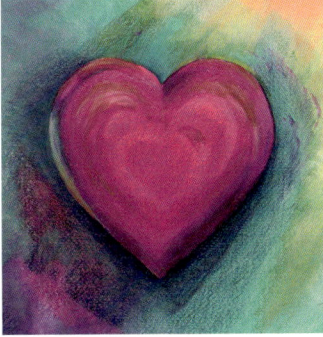

Mental Illness

Mental, or psychological, illnesses and disorders occur in or relate to the mind. Unlike physical health problems and medical conditions, there are no laboratory tests such as blood and urine analyses or x rays to help physicians and other mental health professionals to diagnose mental illnesses. Instead they must rely on listening carefully to patients' complaints and observing their behavior to assess their moods, motivations, and thinking.

Concepts and understanding of mental health and mental illness have changed throughout history and varied from one culture to another. For the most part mental health was not well defined; it was simply the absence of mental illness. Mental illness included a wide range of problems but was generally understood as behavior that was abnormal or different from the majority of society.

In a world in which cultural and social differences are abundant, within and between countries and continents, it is very difficult to define "normal" behavior and "abnormal" behavior. The symptoms associated with mental illness also varied over time and across cultures. For example, some cultures revered people who claimed to speak directly with god(s) and considered them spiritual leaders in their communities. In other cultures might such behavior may be interpreted as a symptom of mental illness.

Another way of identifying abnormal behavior is personal distress and the degree of an individual's suffering. For example, does a person's grief over something fall outside the scope of the expected or "normal" level of grief or is it exceeding the average time it takes for an individual to recover from the grief? Another factor in determining abnormality of behavior is whether a person's response to a situation is unexpected. For example, thirst is an expected response to not drinking enough fluids, but becoming emotionally distraught over thirst would be an unexpected response.

Finally, disability and dysfunction are also used to assess an individual's wellbeing. For example, someone with an irrational fear of elevators

Words to Know

Adaptive behavior: The ways in which people adjust to new situations.

Affect: The expression of emotion or feelings displayed to others through facial expressions, hand gestures, voice tone, and other emotional signs.

Affectations: Artificial attitudes or behaviors.

Anhedonia: The inability to experience pleasure.

Antipsychotic drugs: Drugs that reduce psychotic behavior, often having negative long-term side effects.

Anxiety: An abnormal and overwhelming sense of worry and fear that is often accompanied by physical reaction.

Attention-Deficit / Hyperactivity Disorder (ADHD): A disorder that involves difficulty concentrating and overall inattentiveness.

Autism: A developmental disorder marked by the inability to relate socially and by severe withdrawal from reality. Language limitations and the extreme desire for things to remain the same are common symptoms.

Coexisting: Occurring at the same time.

Compulsion: Habitual behaviors or mental acts an individual is driven to perform in order to reduce stress and anxiety brought on by obsessive thoughts.

Correlation: The relation of two or more things that is not naturally expected.

Delusions: False or irrational beliefs people hold despite proof that their beliefs are untrue.

Depression: A disorder marked by constant feelings of sadness, emptiness, and irritability as well as a lack of pleasure in activities.

Down syndrome: A form of mental retardation due to an extra chromosome present at birth, often accompanied by physical characteristics, such as sloped eyes.

Dysfunction: The inability to function properly.

Dyslexia: A disorder that centers on difficulties with word recognition.

Empathy: Understanding of another's situation and feelings.

Enuresis: The inability to control one's bladder while sleeping at night; bed-wetting.

or heights or insects might not be able to participate in daily activities or may experience a great deal of personal distress because of this fear.

This chapter describes a variety of major mental conditions and disorders. Some are deep-rooted mental illnesses, such as schizophrenia; others are more easily treated, such as learning disorders. Most mental disorders are treatable and, like many physical disorders, are not the result of something a person has done to influence the development of the disorder. Mental illness, like physical disease, can and does strike

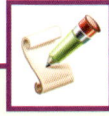

Genetic: Something present in the genes that is inherited from a person's biological parents.

Hallucinations: The perception of things when they aren't really present.

Humane: Marked by compassion or sympathy for other people or creatures.

Intelligence quotient (IQ): A standardized measure of a person's mental ability as compared to those in his or her age group.

Internalized: To incorporate something into one's self.

Irrational: Lacking reason or understanding.

Learning disorders: Developmental problems relating to speech, academic, or language skills that are not linked to a physical disorder or mental retardation.

Obsessions: Repeating thoughts, impulses, or mental images that are irrational and uncontrollable.

Phobia: A form of an anxiety disorder that involves intense and illogical fear of an object or situation.

Physiological: Relating to the functions and activities of life on a biological level.

Post-traumatic stress disorder (PTSD): Reliving trauma and anxiety related to an event that occurred earlier.

Remorse: Feelings of sadness and regret stemming from guilt over past actions.

Residential treatment: Treatment that takes place in a facility in which patients reside.

Savant: A person with extensive knowledge in a very specific area.

Schizophrenia: A chronic psychological disorder marked by scattered, disorganized thoughts, confusion, and delusions.

Social norms: Standard practices that are largely accepted by society.

Somatogenesis: Originating in the body, as opposed to the mind.

Stressor: Something (for example, an event) that causes physical or emotional stress.

Suicide: Taking one's own life.

Tic: A quirk of behavior or speech that happens frequently and repeatedly.

Tourette's Disorder: A disorder marked by the presence of multiple motor tics and at least one vocal tic, as well as compulsions and hyperactivity.

people from all walks of life. And just as treatment for physical ailments has improved markedly over time, so has the diagnosis and treatment of mental illness.

Childhood Disorders

The classification of abnormal behavior in childhood depends greatly on development in terms of behavior considered normal for a child at a certain age. Because children develop at different rates, only a mental

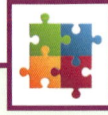

The DSM, IV

DSM-IV (*Diagnostic and Statistical Manual of Mental Disorders*) is an encyclopedia of mental disorders. This guide, which expands on the *ICD-10* (the *International Statistical Classification of Diseases, Injuries, and Causes of Death* lists all medical diseases and included abnormal behavior), is the most widely used psychiatric reference in the world and catalogs more than 300 mental disorders.

Controversy still exists around the DSM because much of it is based on the definitions and categorization of mental illnesses. Looking at past versions of the *DSM* shows that the definitions of mental illnesses have changed from one edition to another. People diagnosed with a specific mental disorder based on diagnostic criteria in one edition might no longer be considered mentally ill according to the next edition. Critics of the *DSM*, which has expanded to more than 10 times its original length from its first edition in 1952, claim that diseases are added randomly by the APA and that even though some entries represent changing ideas about mental health and illness, others are politically motivated. For example, homosexuality was once considered a mental illness, but in the 21st century, largely in response to changing societal attitudes, it is no longer considered an illness. With each new edition of the DSM, efforts are made to address these concerns.

The DSM IV employs a multiaxial system of classification to rate an individual on five health professional can make the distinction between appropriate and inappropriate behavior. Also, childhood disorders can be a sensitive subject because parents and children may fear the social stigma (shame) that often comes with a diagnosis or "label". Children and adolescents strive for acceptance, and any indication of being different or being separated into "special" classes can have devastating effects on a child's self-esteem. Children and teens also may worry about how their peers will react to a label or special accommodations for a learning disorder.

Attention-Deficit / Hyperactivity Disorder Attention-deficit / hyperactivity disorder (ADHD) is a disorder that involves difficulty concentrating and overall inattentiveness. ADHD affects people of all ages but is usually diagnosed in childhood. This condition has received a great deal of attention in the media because there has been a marked increase in the number of diagnoses of this disorder by mental health practitioners in recent years. No longer seen just as a problem of hyperactivity, or excessive activity, ADHD also encompasses a child's difficulty in concentrating on tasks at hand. While most children have notoriously different levels. This is done to ensure that a wide array of possibilities and factors are considered when diagnosing a patient. Axis I includes all categories of mental disorders except personality disorders and mental retardation. These two categories comprise Axis II. Axis III covers medical conditions that are important to understanding a mental disorder, such as Alzheimer disease. Axis IV includes problems or events that can affect the diagnosis, treatment, and outlook of a mental disorder (such as a death in the family, problems at work or school, and even issues such as living in an unsafe neighborhood). Axis V involves the use of the Global Assessment of Functioning (GAF) Scale, which mental health professionals use to assess how well an individual is functioning on a scale of 1 to 100. Taken together, these axes help mental health professionals arrive at a diagnosis

that takes into account all aspects of an individual's life and personality.

The fifth edition of the *DSM*, *DSM-V*, is scheduled for release in May 2013. The diagnostic criteria for the fifth edition emphasize gender and cultural sensitivity and how gender, race, and ethnicity may influence the diagnosis of mental illness. Furthermore, the fifth edition includes new categories for learning disorders and a single category, autism spectrum disorders, that contains a variety of diagnoses such as Asperger disorder (which affects the ability to socialize and communicate with others), childhood disintegrative disorder (a serious loss or absence of social, communication, and other skills), and pervasive developmental disorder (a group of disorders that are characterized by delays in the development of socialization and communication skills).

short spans of attention, children with ADHD have increased difficulty controlling their level of activity and attention, particularly in situations that call for maintaining a certain degree of composure, such as in the classroom or in public places like restaurants.

ADHD makes it difficult for sufferers to sit still or even to stop talking. When they are called upon to be quiet and remain seated, they may squirm, fidget, tap their hands, swing their feet and legs, and make noise. The diagnosis is often difficult to make, because most children are full of energy, particularly during times of play. However, children suffering from ADHD are disorganized, bossy, and ill mannered more often than the average child. Children with ADHD have trouble socializing, are often unable to make friends, and suffer from low self-esteem. Left untreated ADHD can leave children unable to cope in school or socially, and the disorder may lead to depression, conduct disorder, or substance abuse.

Because of the increased prevalence of this diagnosis in recent years, there has been the suggestion that children who are appropriately energetic, hard to handle, or suffering from a conduct disorder (see below)

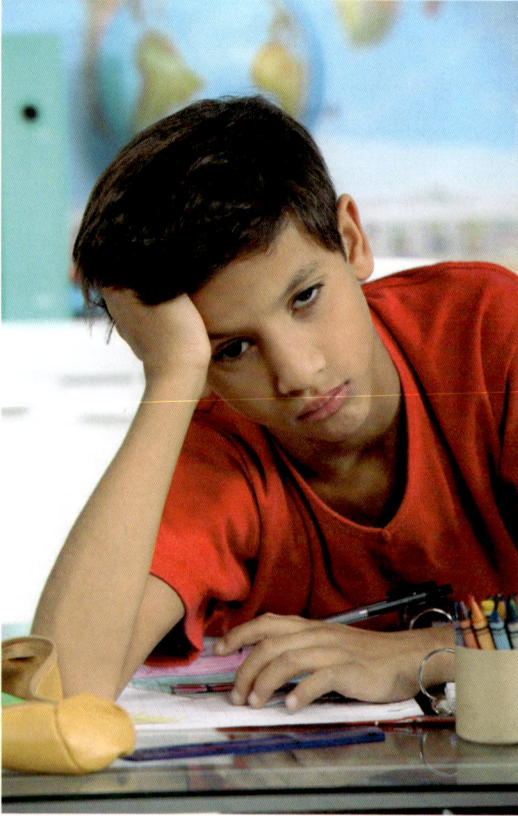

Attention-deficit / hyperactivity disorder can make it difficult for some kids to concentrate in school. © AUREMAR/ SHUTTERSTOCK.COM.

are mistakenly given a diagnosis of ADHD. On the other hand, some experts fear that some children with ADHD may not be diagnosed because parents and teachers mistakenly believe that they just have emotional or disciplinary problems.

Symptoms. According to the National Institute of Mental Health (NIMH), the symptoms of ADHD include inattentive behavior such as lack of attention to details; difficulty paying attention in school or at play; not paying attention when being spoken to; not following through on instructions or failure to finish things; and disorganization, forgetfulness, and losing or misplacing important things. They also have symptoms of hyperactivity such as fidgeting excessively; difficulty playing quietly; and excessive talking as well as symptoms of impulsivity such as difficulty in waiting for their turns and a tendency to interrupt others. To be diagnosed with the disorder, a child must have symptoms for 6 or more months and to a degree that is greater than other children of the same age.

Causes. Although there is no known single cause for ADHD, there are theories about why certain children develop ADHD. Results of twin studies suggest that ADHD is inherited and ADHD often runs in families. Environmental toxins, such as an expectant mother's cigarette smoking or alcohol use may be linked to risk of developing ADHD. Food additives, like artificial color or flavors, and early exposure in infancy and preschool to high levels of lead from paint or plumbing in old buildings may contribute.

Treatments. Treatments do not cure ADHD; they aim to reduce the symptoms of ADHD and improve functioning. Treatments include medication, different types of psychotherapy such as such as behavior modification, education, or a combination of different treatments. Some people also use special diets, nutritional supplements, or biofeedback to teach people affected by ADHD to sharpen their focus and improve their concentration. The most common treatment is the use of a prescription drug "stimulant."

Children and teens with ADHD actually feel and act calmer when given stimulants. There are ADHD medications that are non-stimulants that also help to reduce symptoms for many children. Sometimes children have to try more than one medication or different doses to find the one that works best and produces the fewest side effects. The most common side effects of stimulant drugs are decreased appetite and sleep problems.

Conduct Disorder Although conduct disorders cover a wide array of "bad" behaviors, the diagnosis is made when an individual exhibits inappropriate behaviors that violate the basic rights of other people. These are behaviors that fall outside the scope of normal childhood pranks and mischief; rather, conduct disorder includes behavior that is often vicious, and sufferers typically display no remorse (regret or guilt for having done something wrong), something that links conduct disorder to antisocial personality disorder or psychopathy.

Children or adolescents with conduct disorder are aggressive. They may fight, sexually assault, or behave cruelly to people or animals. Since lying, stealing, vandalism, truancy, and substance abuse are common behaviors of teens with conduct disorders, adults, social service agencies, and the criminal justice system often view such young people as "bad" rather than mentally ill.

In addition to the dysfunctional behaviors they exhibit, people with conduct disorders do not have a great deal of empathy (understanding of other people's feelings). Sufferers also may mistakenly believe others are behaving aggressively toward them when they are not. Although young people with conduct disorders might seem to have tough exterior, they may in fact have low self-esteem. Recklessness, angry outbursts, and the tendency to get easily frustrated are also common symptoms.

Children and adolescents with conduct disorders have trouble in many areas of their lives. Their schoolwork suffers, as do their relationships with parents, teachers, and peers.

Symptoms. The DSM splits conduct disorder symptoms into four categories: aggression toward people and animals (bullying, fighting, use of weapons, physical cruelty to both, stealing, and forced sexual contact); destruction of property (setting fires and destroying property deliberately through another method); deceitfulness or theft (breaking and entering, lying, covert stealing [e.g., forging a check]); and serious violations of rules (staying out past curfew at a young age, running away

Children and teens with ADHD need extra help getting and staying organized. Maintaining a schedule with the same routine every day can help. Organizing clothing, books, toys, backpacks and school supplies makes it easier to find things. Using notebooks, folders and organizers for schoolwork can help students prevent misplacing important assignments.

from home, and cutting school). The American Academy of Child and Adolescent Psychiatry describes the antisocial behaviors that suggest a diagnosis of conduct disorder. These actions and behaviors include:

- bullies, threatens, or intimidates others
- often initiates physical fights
- use of a weapon such as a bat, brick, knife, or gun that could cause serious physical harm
- physical cruelty to people or animals
- steals from victims while confronting them
- engages in coercive or forced sexual activity
- deliberately sets fires with the intention to cause damage
- deliberately destroys property
- has broken into a building, house, or car
- lies to obtain goods or favors or to avoid obligations
- steals items without confronting a victim
- often stays out at night despite parental objections
- runs away from home
- often absent without cause from school

Causes. Just as with ADHD, there is no known single cause for conduct disorders, but there are theories that explain why certain children develop conduct disorders. One theory is that conduct disorders may be inherited ailments. Another possibility is that there is a lack of moral awareness in the family of origin of a person suffering from conduct disorder. In general, children learn what is right and wrong and refrain from breaking the boundaries of decency because they have been taught that it is wrong to hurt others. If, for whatever reason, these lessons are not learned in the home, a conduct disorder, or even more serious psychological problems, could develop. Furthermore, a child may witness disordered conduct from his or her parents and learn aggressive, improper behavior.

Other researchers propose that children prone to developing conduct disorder may have flawed thinking processes. That is, very aggressive children may perceive an otherwise harmless event (for instance, being last in a line), as an offense, place unusual importance on the event, and hold a grudge because of the occurrence. Some known risk factors that increase the likelihood of developing conduct disorders include a family history of mental illness, especially parents with serious mental disorders; separation from parents with no consistent caregiver; early institutionalization; family neglect, abuse, or violence; parental marital conflict; large family size; overcrowding; and poverty. In these circumstances children may lack feelings of attachment to their parents or families, and later, to the community. Eventually they express these feelings of alienation (isolation and separation) by behaving with disregard for society's rules and values. Some mental health professionals describe people with conduct disorders as appearing to lack a "moral compass."

Treatments. The most successful treatments of conduct disorders involve treating not only the child or teen (or adult) but also those around him or her as well (family and, in some cases, friends). Cognitive behavioral therapy, in which a therapist helps a patient become aware of maladaptive thinking and flawed belief systems and helps change beliefs that can interfere with healthy living, may also improve behavior,

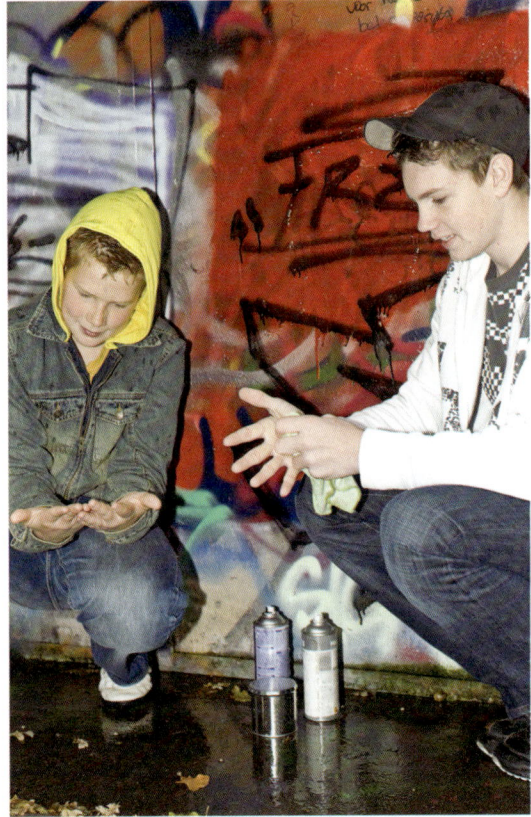

Many adolescents and teens play pranks or get into mischief, but repeated antisocial behaviors, including vandalism and increasingly violent behaviors, may be symptoms of a conduct disorder. © COREPICS VOF/SHUTTERSTOCK.COM.

as can teaching children moral reasoning skills. While therapy can reduce some antisocial behavior, living with a child or teen with a conduct disorder stresses the entire family. Support programs train parents how to positively reinforce appropriate behaviors and how to strengthen the emotional bonds between parents and children. Identifying and taking action with children at risk for conduct disorders to improve their social interactions and prevent school failure can reduce some of the harmful long-term consequences of conduct disorder.

Oppositional Defiant Disorder Children often disobey their parents or teachers, particularly when they are extremely young, as a way of asserting their independence. However, when a child consistently is disobedient, disrespectful, hostile, and defiant toward parents, teachers, and other figures of authority for a period of six months, the child may be diagnosed with oppositional defiant disorder (ODD), a disorder that is not uncommon. Stubbornness and an unwillingness to deal rationally with others when there is disagreement are also signs of ODD.

Because defiant behavior is a common development in both very young children and teenagers, it is cautioned that mental health practitioners make this diagnosis very carefully. Interestingly, more boys tend to suffer from ODD than girls do in the years before puberty; however, when adolescence arrives, both girls and boys are diagnosed at about the same rate.

Children and teens with ODD argue with peers and adults, lose their tempers, refuse to follow rules, behave annoyingly on purpose, blame others for their own mistakes, and are angry, spiteful, and vindictive. Their behaviors often distance them from family and peers and cause problems at school.

Some mental health professionals consider ODD a "gateway condition" to conduct disorder and believe that the progression to conduct disorder can be prevented with timely treatment. Treatment for ODD often involves cognitive therapy and operant conditioning therapy featuring a system of rewards.

While ODD often shares similarities with both ADHD and conduct disorder, there are differences. Conduct disorder usually manifests itself in physical violence, while ODD usually does not. ODD differs from ADHD in that the "bratty" behavior seen in ODD seems to be conscious and planned, while ADHD sufferers seem to be unable control their impulses or actions when exhibiting such behaviors.

Learning Disorders Learning disorders refer to developmental problems relating to speech, motor, and academic or language skills that are not linked to a physical disorder or mental retardation. The presence of a learning disability is not a reflection of a person's intelligence. In fact, people with learning disabilities often have average or above-average intelligence, but there is a problem in development or information processing that prevents them from understanding complex ideas. Most often, parents and teachers become aware of learning disorders through a child's results on standardized academic tests administered by the school. Because many learning disorders run in families, it is believed that they may be inherited, particularly the reading disorder called dyslexia.

The treatment of learning disorders focuses on instruction in the area in which there are problems. The most effective programs are those that give children a chance to make small steps toward progress, which can help to restore their self-esteem and confidence.

Learning disorders are described by the difficulties they create: reading disorder, mathematics disorder, and disorder of written expression; there is also a general diagnosis (learning disorder, not otherwise specified) that covers any combination of these problems. Between 10–20% of children and teens have a learning disorder, language disorder, or both.

Reading Disorder. One developmental reading disorder is commonly known as dyslexia (pronounced dis-LEX-ee-a). Dyslexia comes from the Greek words "dys" (meaning poor or inadequate) and "lexis" (which refers to words or language). Dyslexia is a disorder that centers on difficulties with word recognition. Sufferers most often add, omit, or transpose (change the sequence of) letters in a word (for example, mistaking "sing" for "sign" or "left" for "felt"). All of these symptoms reveal themselves in problems with reading aloud, comprehending what is read, and spelling words correctly. Dyslexia can also affect mathematical skills, causing the person to add, omit, or transpose numbers. Research shows that people with dyslexia process information in a different area of the brain than those who do not have this learning disorder.

Disorder of Written Expression. Disorder of written expression centers on problems with writing skills. This disorder, also known as dysgraphia, makes the act of writing difficult and this can affect many areas of academics, as can a reading disorder. Children, teens, and adults with dysgraphia may find it difficult to organize letters, numbers, and words on a line or page. Poor handwriting, as well as difficulty with punctuation, grammar, and spelling, is common. While many young people may have difficulties with some or all of these things, this diagnosis is made when the problem is so severe that it interferes with academic achievement.

Mathematics Disorder. Between six and seven percent of children and teens have a mathematical learning disorder (also known as dyscalculia). While math can be difficult for many people, some children have difficulties that go beyond the normal scope. The problem can be as serious as someone being unable to recognize mathematical symbols and numbers to having difficulty following the proper steps to solve a mathematical equation. The degree of the difficulty is the key to making a diagnosis of mathematics disorder.

Just because someone has a learning disorder doesn't mean they won't be successful. Many very intelligent, talented and successful people have overcome learning disabilities to achieve great things, from Leonardo da Vinci and Albert Einstein to Keira Knightley, Justin Timberlake, Michael Phelps, and Solange Knowles.

Mental Retardation Mental retardation is a condition of below-normal mental ability or intelligence due to disease, injury, or genetic defect. It is generally diagnosed before age 18. Parents are often the first to recognize mental retardation when their children's motor, language, and self-help skills appear to be developing more slowly than others their age. The degree of mental retardation varies from severely or profoundly impaired to very mild or borderline retardation. Although serious difficulty adjusting to new situations and very slow intellectual progress make it easier to identify children with moderate to severe mental retardation, children with mild mental retardation may not be identified until they enter school.

Most people have an intelligence quotient (IQ) between 70 and 130, with the majority of the population having IQs between 85 and 115. (IQ is the measure of intelligence based on intelligence tests and the intelligence of the general population.) People with some degree of mental retardation have IQs below 70 and as low as 20. Along with this low level of intelligence, people with mental retardation have trouble with adaptive behavior or functioning. They may lack skills such as dressing, responding appropriately in social interactions, and understanding abstract concepts like time and money.

Symptoms The symptoms of mental retardation vary depending on the degree of the disorder but may include continued infant-like behavior, decreased or very slow learning, inability to meet predetermined markers of intellectual development, inability to perform in school, and lack of curiosity. People with mild mental retardation may be quiet, withdrawn, and lack interest in things while those with severe mental retardation never progress beyond infant-like behavior.

Causes. The most common causes of mental retardation are infections present at birth or occurring shortly after birth such as encephalitis (swelling of the brain) and meningococcal meningitis (swelling of the lining around the brain or spinal cord); chromosomal abnormalities such as Down syndrome; genetic and other inherited disorders such as Tay-Sachs disease; metabolic problems such as poorly regulated blood sugar levels or Reye syndrome (sudden, acute brain damage most often seen in young children); severe malnutrition; toxic exposures pre-birth such as exposure to alcohol, cocaine, amphetamines, and other drugs or lead poisoning; and trauma before and after birth such as severe head injury or lack of oxygen to the brain before, during, or immediately after birth.

Down syndrome usually causes people to have moderate to severe retardation. Furthermore, Down syndrome sufferers share certain physical characteristics that have become hallmarks of the disorder, including oval, upward-slanting eyes; fine straight hair; and a stocky build and short stature. Often, there is no identifiable biological cause for mental retardation, especially in the cases of mildly or moderately mentally retarded individuals.

Treatments. Treatment aims to help each person to grow, develop, and maintain the highest level of functioning possible to realize their full potential. Treatment of mental retardation varies depending on the degree of retardation. Residential treatment, that is, treatment in live-in homes or facilities, is very popular. Sometimes a patient will develop enough skills to move into a group home, which features a home-like setting and living with people at similar levels of functioning. Some people with mental retardation benefit from treatments such as operant conditioning and cognitive behavioral therapies. It also is very important that these vulnerable individuals be treated with compassion and protected so they may lead comfortable, happy lives.

There are four major diagnoses relating directly to mental retardation:

Mild Mental Retardation. The IQ range for this diagnosis is between 50 and 55 to 70. Frequently these individuals are not diagnosed as mentally retarded until later in their development because they are usually able to learn at a sixth-grade level. People who are mildly mentally retarded can usually hold jobs and often marry and successfully raise children. More than three-quarters of mentally retarded people have been diagnosed in this category.

Moderate Mental Retardation. Ten percent of the mentally retarded are diagnosed with an IQ range of 35–40 to 50–55. Physical problems, including brain damage, are often present, and tasks such as running or grasping things can be extremely difficult. Many people in this category live with their families or in supervised group homes with a great deal of success.

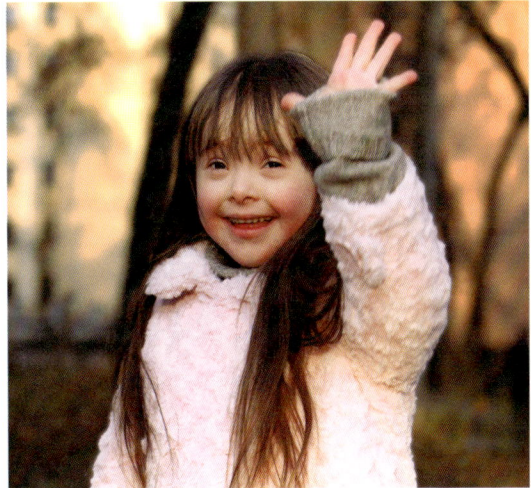

According to the Centers for Disease Control, about one in every 691 babies in the United States is born with Down syndrome, which is the result of an extra chromosome. Though cognitive abilities of those with Down syndrome vary widely, with the proper support of family and specialized education opportunities, many children with Down syndrome integrate successfully into society. © DENIS KUVAEV/ SHUTTERSTOCK.COM.

Severe Mental Retardation. Approximately three to four percent of individuals with mental retardation are at this level, with an IQ range of 20–25 to 35–40. Birth defects are often present, and communication skills are limited. Although they may be able to perform certain tasks under supervision, often they are unable to function independently in any capacity.

Profound Mental Retardation. One to two percent of people with mental retardation have IQs falling below 20–25. These individuals require supervision for their entire lives. Because of related medical problems and disabilities, people with this diagnosis often have a short life span.

Autism Autism is a group of developmental disorders, which taken together is called autism spectrum disorder (ASD). The term spectrum explains that there is a wide range and variety of symptoms, skills, and disabilities among children with a diagnosis of ASD. Some children are very mildly troubled by their symptoms and others are severely disabled. The DSM-IV has five disorders within the autism spectrum—classic autism, Asperger syndrome, pervasive developmental disorder not otherwise specified (PDD-NOS), Rett syndrome (children develop normally for 6–18 months before they backslide and autism-like symptoms begin), and childhood disintegrative disorder (children develop normally until age three or four and then lose their language and social skills). However, the DSM-V will no longer consider Asperger syndrome as a diagnosis. Instead, it will be considered part of the autism spectrum.

In the NBC series *Parenthood*, actor Max Burkholder plays Max Braverman, a teenager with Asperger syndrome. For many of the show's viewers, this is the first time they have seen the challenges a young person with Asperger syndrome faces in family life, at school, and making friends. This portrayal helps to improve awareness and understanding of autism spectrum disorders.

Autism spectrum disorders are marked by the inability to relate socially to others and by severe withdrawal from reality. Language limitations and the extreme desire for things to remain constant are common traits of autism. Autistic children and adults seem to "look through" people and very often avoid eye contact. More often than not, they are unresponsive to touch and are unable to accept and display affection. An interest in ritual and repetitive body movements, such as rocking back and forth, and repeating of certain words or phrases, are also usually present. In many cases, speech is absent and, when it is present, autistic individuals are often unable to hold a conversation with others. In some cases, people with autism may form strong attachments to inanimate (nonliving) objects, such as keys or even a refrigerator.

Children with ASD develop differently from their age peers. Even as babies they may become unusually focused on certain objects, rarely

The Temple Grandin Story

There are people with ASD who have managed to become fully functional adults. One woman, Temple Grandin, Ph.D. (1947–), was diagnosed with autism at the age of three. Her case has been documented by neurologist Dr. Oliver Sacks, and she has written two autobiographical books. Grandin managed to learn how to speak by age six and went on to earn her doctoral degree in animal science, to run her own business, and teach courses at Colorado State University. However, for all of her academic and professional achievements, she still remains in awe of people and human relations, calling herself an "observer" rather than a participant in the social realm of life. While she has managed to overcome many of the negative traits of autism, such as violent rages and acting out impulsively and seemingly without reason, she has been unable to bridge the gap between herself and others on an emotional level. Dr. Sacks noted that while Grandin is able to converse at length about intellectual matters, she lacks many standard social graces (manners).

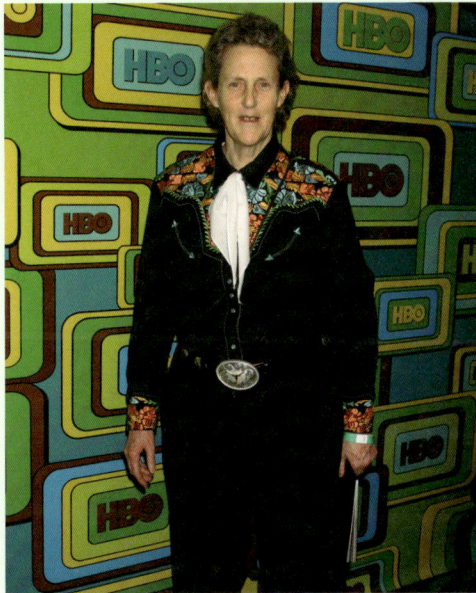

Temple Grandin arrives at an HBO Golden Globe party in 2011 for an opening of the movie about her life starring Claire Danes as Grandin. © HELGA ESTEB/SHUTTERSTOCK.COM.

make eye contact, and do not begin to coo and babble and interact socially. Other children appear to develop normally until age two or three and then suddenly withdraw and even backslide in terms of development, losing some of the language and other skills they had already mastered.

Children with ASD may not respond to their names or other verbal attempts to get their attention, and they may only slowly develop gestures, such as pointing to show things to others. Their pace of language development is slow, and some are only able to communicate using pictures or their own sign language. Many children and adolescents with ASD are unable to combine words into meaningful sentences and repeat words or phrases that they hear over and over.

Savants

In his book, *The Man Who Mistook His Wife for a Hat*, renowned neurologist Dr. Oliver Sacks (1933–) described the savant qualities possessed by some autistic people. For example, while speaking with autistic twins at the hospital in which they lived, a box of matches fell on the floor. Moments later, both twins shrieked, "111." Dr. Sacks was confused until he painstakingly counted the matches to discover there were, indeed, 111. When he pressed the twins about how they knew how many matches there were on the floor, they said that they simply "saw" the number and looked at him in bewilderment over the fact that he hadn't.

Often those with ASD make repetitive motions or display unusual behaviors. For example, some children may repeatedly flap their arms or walk in specific patterns, while others may tap repeatedly on a table or other surface. Children with ASD also are likely to have overly focused interests. They may prefer to arrange their toys rather than play with them. Because order is very important to them, they may be very upset if someone accidentally moves one of their toys. Children and teens with ASD often become obsessed with learning everything they can about very specific topics like locomotives, bus schedules, or insects. They are particularly interested in numbers, symbols, and science.

Children with ASD do not like, or adapt well to, change so they tend do best with routine in their daily activities and surroundings. They are frequently inflexible and may insist on eating the same sandwich for lunch every day or taking the same exact route home from school. Even very slight changes in their routines can be so upsetting that they are overcome by anger or frustration.

Another aspect of autism is that while many suffering from the disorder are mentally retarded to some degree (approximately 80 percent), they also may display almost incredible skill in other areas, such as mathematics. This facet of autism has prompted the use of the term "idiot savant." A savant is someone with detailed knowledge in a specialized field, such as math or science. Some people suffering from autism may have exceptional memories or a profound physical grace. Others with autism may, however, exhibit awkward physical affectations, movements and posture and may not possess any outstanding, savant-like abilities.

Causes. Autism has its origins in biology, and studies of twins indicate that ASD may be genetic in origin. In the majority of cases, when one identical twin has ASD, the other twin also has ASD. When one sibling has ASD, the other siblings have 35 times the normal risk of developing ASD. Researchers are identifying the specific genes that may increase the risk for ASD. They also are looking at environmental factors that may affect certain genes.

Treatment. Treatment for autism is not always effective. However, operant conditioning and modeling have proven to be successful in enabling parents to, at the very least, bring their children into social situations without the children acting out. Some therapists have had success in using intense behavioral therapy as well. Depending on where people fall on the autism spectrum and the skills they are able to master, some people with ASD may be able to live independently as adults. Others will live at home with their parents or in supervised group homes where they can get some help with the activities of daily living such as preparing meals, shopping, and cleaning house. People with severe ASD who require constant supervision may live in long-term care facilities.

Tourette Syndrome Usually diagnosed before age 18, Tourette syndrome is a neurological disorder (a disorder of the brain) that causes multiple motor tics and at least one vocal tic (a tic is a quirk of behavior or speech that happens frequently and repeatedly). Examples of tics include frequent eye blinking, throat clearing, shoulder shrugging, sniffing, repeating words or sounds over and over, or, less frequently, coprolalia (repeatedly saying obscenities). The diagnosis of Tourette syndrome is made when symptoms occur for more than a year, without a lapse in symptoms of more than three months in a row. In addition, the condition must have a negative effect in at least one area of functioning—in the person's social, educational, or professional life. More common in males than females, Tourette syndrome usually begins between the ages of three and nine.

Symptoms. The symptoms of Tourette syndrome range from obsessions and compulsions to hyperactivity, social discomfort, and depression. Social problems and depression may stem from embarrassment over sufferers' inability to control their actions. Exaggerated behaviors not uncommon to Tourette, such as head banging, knee bending, head jerking, and picking the skin, can cause injury and/or illness.

Causes. Tourette syndrome is an inherited disorder. While not all individuals who inherit the predisposition toward Tourette will develop the disorder, 70 percent of females and 99 percent of men carrying the genes will develop it or a milder tic disorder.

Treatments. Tourette syndrome is often treated with prescription drugs, which can help to lessen the presence of tics and other symptoms. Behavioral treatments also may help people to control tics.

Bed-Wetting

For many children, nighttime enuresis, or bed-wetting, is an embarrassing and painful problem. The inability to control one's bladder while sleeping is stressful, and children with this problem may suffer from low self-esteem. Enuresis is not diagnosed until a child is at least five years old (the age by which most children have been toilet-trained). At age five, about seven percent of boys and three percent of girls are enuretic. Furthermore, the majority of children with enuresis have always had problems with bladder control during the night (they are called primary enuretics); far fewer are considered secondary enuretics, meaning they were once able to control their bladders but have lost that ability.

A variety of factors have been blamed for bed-wetting. There is a strong genetic link for bed-wetting (if a parent wet the bed, the child is much more likely to do so). Bed-wetting is more common in boys than girls, and children with ADHD are more likely to have this problem. Certain medical conditions cause enuresis, such as urinary tract infections, kidney disease, diabetes, sleep apnea (a condition in which breathing is interrupted during sleep (in children this is often caused by enlarged tonsils or adenoids). It also may be caused by the child's bladder being too small to hold all the urine produced during the night or by a hormonal imbalance—some children do not produce enough anti-diuretichormone (ADH)—this hormone slows the production of urine at night. Some therapists believe that stress may be a cause of bed-wetting. Moving, starting a new school, or family stress such as illness of divorce may trigger this problem.

Most children outgrow bed-wetting. When treatment is needed, many children treated using principles of classical conditioning learn to stop bed-wetting. Drs. O. H. Mowrer and W. M. Mowrer developed a moisture alarm based on these principles. The bell-and-pad apparatus involves a pad that, when moisture hits it, sounds a bell, waking the child and prompting him to go to the bathroom to finish urinating. Prescription medicine is also effective in ending episodes of bed-wetting but is only effective when it is being used; when the children stop taking the drugs, the bed-wetting returns.

Stuttering Most people have heard someone stutter. People who stutter may find it hard to start a new word, make some words sound longer than they should, repeat words or parts of words, or get nervous and tense when they have to speak. They may even tremble as they try to speak. Stuttering is a disturbance in verbal fluency of speech; for example, a stutterer might repeat whole words several times before being able to move on to the next word in the sentence ("I want to go-go-go-go to the movies."). Another sign may be a person's consistent difficulty in pronouncing certain consonants, or having long pauses between words in a sentence.

Stuttering is frustrating because, like Tourette syndrome, it separates people from others by hampering easy communication. It can also affect learning, as a child may be embarrassed to ask or answer questions in class because of fear of classmates' teasing. Furthermore, stuttering can become worse when people are nervous, which can prevent stutterers from answering difficult questions or doing any type of public speaking.

Boys are three times more likely to stutter than girls. Most children outgrow or overcome stuttering as they get older. Stuttering is uncommon among adults—less than 1 percent of adults stutter.

Speech-language pathologists perform therapy with stutterers to help them overcome the disorder. Many people have overcome stuttering and gone on to become successful and famous. Among them are actors James Earl Jones, Emily Blunt, Nicole Kidman, Nicholas Brendon, Bruce Willis, and Eric Roberts as well as musicians John Lee Hooker, B.B. King, Nancy Wilson, Francois Goudreault, and Marc Anthony.

Mood Disorders

Mood disorders cause a disturbance in mood (state of mind) and include depression and bipolar disorders. Mood disorders can be devastating. Depending on their severity, they can emotionally paralyze people, leaving them unable to work or attend classes or even enjoy the most basic things. Mood disorders can also disrupt appetite and sleep patterns and sufferers' sense of well being.

Major Depression Major depression, the condition of feeling deep and constant sadness, is one of the most common mental disorders. More common in women than in men, depression tends to recur, making it a lifelong battle for some people. Depression, too, has become more common over the last few decades. This may be attributable to social changes that have occurred simultaneously (society moving at a faster pace, people feeling more stressed as life becomes increasingly urbanized, and many institutions—church, family, cultural customs—that once acted as support systems no longer as common). It may also be that people are more aware of the symptoms of depression and are more willing to seek treatment than in the past.

Symptoms. There are several possible symptoms of depression, whether it be a major depressive episode (which lasts approximately up to two weeks) or major depressive disorder (of longer duration with a higher rate of recurrence of the depression). Symptoms can include: constant feelings of sadness, emptiness, or irritability; a lack of pleasure in

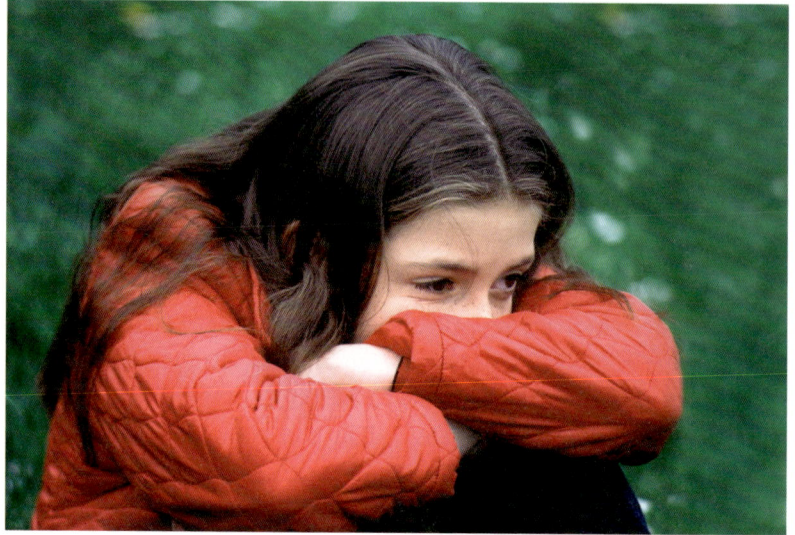

activities, even those that once brought enormous pleasure; a noticeable drop or increase in weight; the inability to sleep; extreme exhaustion; feelings of worthlessness; an inability to make decisions or concentrate on performing tasks; and thoughts of death and suicide.

In order for a diagnosis of depression to be made, none of these symptoms can be caused by drugs or a medical disorder (there are separate categories of depression that are caused by illness or substance abuse). A diagnosis should not be made if an individual is mourning the very recent loss of a loved one. Children who are depressed are similar to adults suffering from depression. They may be teary and sad, lose interest in friends and activities, and become listless, self-critical, and overly sensitive to criticism from others. They feel unloved, helpless, hopeless about the future, and they may think about suicide. Depressed children and adolescents also may be irritable, aggressive, and indecisive. They may have problems concentrating and sleeping and often become careless about their appearance and hygiene. Teens with depression often suffer from other disorders such as anxiety, eating disorders, or substance abuse as well. Without proper treatment, children who are depressed may stay depressed, suffer frequent bouts of depression, or even develop more serious depression as adults.

Causes. Depression may be caused by a combination of genetic, biological, environmental, and psychological factors. One possible factor may be that neurotransmitters (chemicals that brain cells use to communicate) are off balance in people with depression. But it is difficult to prove whether this imbalance is a cause or the result of depression. Research also shows that parts of the brain involved in mood, thinking, sleep, and appetite of people who suffer from depression look different from those of people without depression. But these differences do not explain why the depression occurred or what caused the changes, and again, the changes may be the result rather than the cause of depression. Some types of depression run in families, which suggests a genetic or inherited tendency to develop the disorder. But people without family histories of depression are affected too. Some research suggests that the risk for depression involves several genes acting together with environmental or other factors.

Reactive depression is the most common mental health problem in children and adolescents. It is not considered a mental disorder, and many health professionals consider occasional bouts of reactive depression a completely normal part of growing up and adolescent development. Reactive depression is a brief period of depressed feelings in response to some negative experience, such as a rejection from a boyfriend or girlfriend or getting a failing grade. Sadness or listlessness gets better on its own, without any treatment, in as little as few hours or may last as long as 2 weeks. Generally distraction, such as a change of activity or setting, helps to improve the mood of children or teens that have reactive depression. In children, teens, and adults, painful and difficult events such as the loss of a loved one, a difficult relationship, or other stressful situations may trigger an episode of reactive depression. Other times, depressive episodes may occur without an apparent trigger.

Some psychoanalysts believe that the seeds of depression are sown in early childhood when something goes wrong with one stage of development or another. Cognitive therapists, such as Aaron Beck, believe that an individual battling depression has a faulty perception of the world, tending to view things negatively, and this impacts the person and his or her reactions to different situations later in life, increasing

Overcoming Depression

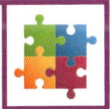

Many people overcome depression to lead happy, successful lives. Even celebrities, who seem to have enchanted lives, can suffer from depression. Many celebrities have spoken publicly about their battles with depression including Jon Hamm, Ashley Judd, Owen Wilson, David Arquette, Catherine Zeta-Jones, Brooke Shields, Winona Ryder, Gwyneth Paltrow, and Demi Lovato. Like many young people with depression, Demi Lovato also acknowledged that she suffered from substance abuse and eating disorders as well.

Suicide: A Deadly Side-Effect of Depression

Suicide is when a person takes his or her own life. Not all people who kill themselves do so solely because of depression. However, many depressed people entertain the thought of ending their lives, attempt to end their lives, or sadly, succeed in ending their lives. Often times, the first sign of a person's depression may be a suicide attempt.

According to the American Psychiatric Association, depression is very common among teenagers and young adults. Studies have shown that teens that are depressed, abusing substances, or acting out on violent feelings are all at high risk for suicide. In fact, among teens and young adults between the ages of 15 and 24, suicide is the third leading cause of death. It is estimated that 5,000 teens commit suicide each year.

Suicide prevention centers around the country offer 24-hour assistance to people in despair and considering suicide. But one of the most important ways to prevent suicide is to be aware of the signs that a depressed or despondent person may be considering taking his or her life. Watching for warning signs of depression or reckless behavior and then helping the person who is depressed to get professional help are crucial steps that can be taken to help prevent suicide. The following are some of the signs that might be cause for concern: talking about wanting to die or kill oneself; looking for ways to kill one self, such as searching online for methods; talking about feeling hopeless, a burden to others, or having no reason to live; use or increasing use of alcohol or drugs; sleep disturbances (sleeping too much or too little), a change in appetite and weight, feelings of restlessness, lack of concentration, withdrawal from friends and activities once considered fun, sudden mood swings, displaying rage or talking about seeking revenge; and feelings of guilt.

susceptibility to developing depression. Behavioral therapists believe that depression may strike individuals who do not have strong social support and whose depression further deepens their isolation from others. There are also those who attribute depression to biological causes, including the possibility that it is inherited or caused by a chemical imbalance in the brain.

Treatments. Depression has been treated with success using cognitive therapy and interpersonal therapy (a therapy that focuses on how a person interacts with others and which instructs him or her how to interact more effectively). Drug therapies have also been used to treat depression. Antidepressants, such as Tofranil and Elavil, as well as Prozac, work on brain chemicals called neurotransmitters, Although these brain chemicals are involved in regulating mood, scientists are not exactly sure how they work. For mild to moderate depression, psychotherapy may be the best choice. However, for severe depression psychotherapy may not be enough to relieve symptoms of depression. Some experts believe that for teens, a combination of antidepressant medication and psychotherapy is the best effective approach for treating severe depression and reducing the chances of it returning.

Bipolar Disorder Bipolar disorders are marked by extreme highs and extreme lows in mood. Similar to depression in that they include the occurrence of major depressive episodes, bipolar disorders are also accompanied by manic episodes or hypomanic episodes. A manic episode is when a person is in an intense emotional state of elation (extreme happiness) and hyperactivity in which he or she is abnormally energetic and talks in an almost stream-of-consciousness way, with ideas and grandiose plans being shared (however implausible they may seem). Examples of other symptoms of a manic episode include an inflated sense of self, a reduced need for sleep, and engaging in reckless activities (for example, irresponsible sexual behavior or excessive spending). A hypomanic episode is similar to a manic episode though not as extreme.

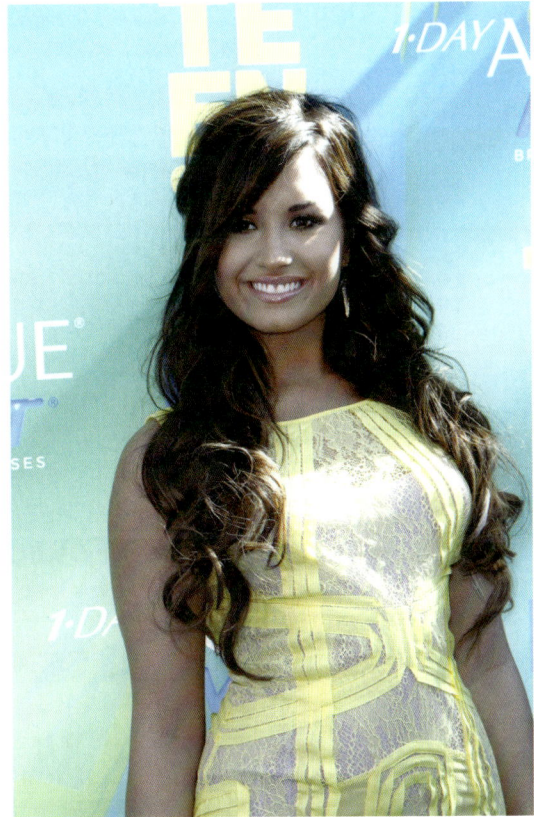

Demi Lovato has been open about her struggles with bipolar disorder. © JOE SEER/ SHUTTERSTOCK.COM.

Adults and adolescents with bipolar disorder alternate between episodes of mania and episodes of depression. The beginning of bipolar illness is usually a depressive episode during adolescence, and manic episodes may not appear for months or even years. During manic episodes adolescents are tireless, overly confident, and tend to have rapid-fire or pressured speech. They may perform tasks and schoolwork quickly and energetically but in a wildly disorganized manner. Manic adolescents may seriously overestimate their capabilities, and the combination of swagger, daring, and loosened inhibitions may cause them to participate in high-risk behaviors, such as vandalism, drug abuse, or unsafe sex.

Bipolar I disorder is marked by severe manic episodes accompanied by major depressive episodes. People with bipolar I disorder need immediate hospital care. Bipolar II disorder is defined by major depressive episodes accompanied by at least one hypomanic episode, but no full-blown manic episodes.

Bipolar depression also differs from major depression, which is also known as unipolar depression, in that it strikes males and females at the same rate. Typically, bipolar depression is treated with medication and counseling. As with major depression, bipolar disorder tends to run in families. Although children with a parent or sibling who has bipolar disorder are four to six times more likely to develop the illness than children without a family history of bipolar disorder, most children with a family history of the disorder will not develop it.

Psychotic Disorders

Psychotic disorders, including schizophrenia, are mental disorders that involve a dramatic impairment in thinking, such that an individual is almost completely out of touch with reality. Most often this means that a person is experiencing hallucinations or having delusions. Hallucinations are the perception of things that aren't present (seeing or hearing things); delusions are false or irrational beliefs that a person holds despite proof that those beliefs are untrue. These qualities make psychotic disorders frightening and mysterious, especially for those afflicted by them.

Schizophrenia The "crazy person" who hears voices, behaves inappropriately, and sometimes ends up as a homeless person, muttering and shouting incomprehensibly, frequently suffers from schizophrenia. Schizophrenia is one of the most severe psychotic disorders. Although treatment helps to relieve many of the symptoms of the disorder, it is a chronic problem, so most sufferers need to be on medication for the rest of their lives. Many people with schizophrenia are unable to resume normal lives; this tragedy is compounded by the fact that schizophrenia often develops when individuals are in their late teens through mid-thirties. This means that some people working toward building a full life find themselves in jeopardy of losing everything they have worked for.

The effects begin slowly and at first are often considered the normal behavioral changes of adolescence. Gradually, voices take over in the person's mind, wiping out reality and directing the person to all kinds of unpredictable behaviors. Suicide attempts are common in the lives of schizophrenics. Many people with schizophrenia turn to drugs in an attempt to escape the torment inflicted by their brains. The NIMH estimated that as many as half of all schizophrenics are also drug abusers. The families of people with schizophrenia also are affected. The disorder can produce frightening and very disruptive behavior, and because people with schizophrenia may not be able to work or take care of themselves, they often must rely on their families for support.

Symptoms. Symptoms of schizophrenia include having scattered, disorganized thoughts. People with schizophrenia lose their train of thought when talking with others, and they may not make sense. They often bring up completely different or entirely unrelated issues, which causes others to become confused. Delusions are another symptom of schizophrenia. Delusions can include anything from a person's belief that others are plotting against him or her; that a person's food is poisoned because someone is trying to kill him; or that another person can read his mind. Hallucinations often accompany delusions as well. Many times, schizophrenics hear strange voices inside their heads. Naturally, this is extremely disturbing and feeds a schizophrenic's fear.

Other symptoms include a lack of motivation to engage in normal daily activities, such as maintaining personal hygiene or doing chores. Also, although schizophrenics will tend to speak, they will have less to say; their conversations may be repetitive and nonsensical. The inability to experience pleasure, known as anhedonia, may also be present, as may problems with a person's affect (an individual's emotional response and demeanor); often times, a schizophrenic's affect may be flat (lacking in emotional response) or inappropriate (for example, laughing upon hearing that someone has died).

Causes. Schizophrenia runs in families. The illness affects 1% of the U.S. population, but about 10% of people who have a parent, brother, or sister with the disorder also will develop it. People with other affected relatives such as aunts, uncles, grandparents, or cousins also develop schizophrenia more often than the general population. The risk is highest for identical twins. If one twin has schizophrenia then the other has a 40–65% chance of developing the disorder.

Chemical imbalances in the brain also may cause or trigger the development of schizophrenia, and the tendency to have a chemical imbalance also may be inherited. Some research suggests that the brain of a schizophrenic manufactures too much dopamine, a chemical vital to normal nerve activity.

Treatments. Schizophrenia may be treated with antipsychotic drugs, such as chlorpromazine (Thorazine) or haloperidol (Haldol), which reduce psychotic symptoms, particularly because hallucinations and delusions can cause schizophrenics to engage in behaviors that make them a risk to themselves and even others around them. But these drugs often produce troubling side effects. Some patients who take these drugs for several years experience side effects such as uncontrollable, spastic muscular contractions and tremors as well as involuntary movements of the face, lips, and tongue (known as *tardive dyskinesia*). Newer antipsychotic medications such as clozapine (Clozaril) and risperidone (Risperidol), olanzepine, (Zyprexa), Aripiprazole (Abilify), Paliperidone (Invega), and quetiapine (Serquel) are as effective and have fewer side effects than previously used medications.

Amber Main looks over some notes before shooting an episode of True Life, *an MTV documentary series that examines issues faced by young people. Main was featured in May 2008, the year after her diagnosis at age 18. The episode, "I Have Schizophrenia," followed Main's struggle to get her academic life in order after battling the mental illness. With the help of medicine and therapy, she was trying to live the life of a typical college student.* © AP IMAGES/THE DAILY PRESS/DAVE BOWMAN.

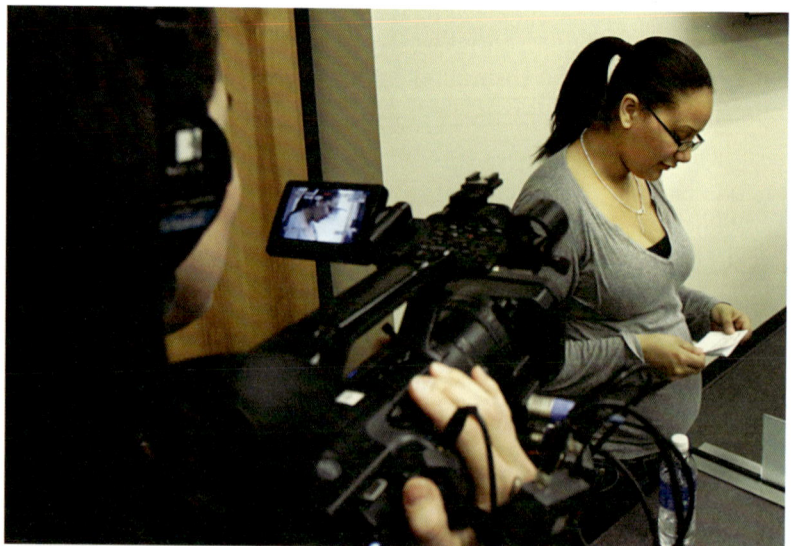

Although medication is usually successful in suppressing symptoms of schizophrenia used alone, it is not enough. Therapy is a necessary ingredient in treatment to help people with schizophrenia accept and cope with their situations and understand the importance of continuing to take medication even if they feel "cured." Patients who receive regular psychosocial treatment are more likely to keep taking their medication, and less likely to be hospitalized. Therapists help patients better understand the problems they may experience and reinforce the importance of staying on medications. Therapy can also be useful in helping the patient's family understand the patient's plight and contribute to helping manage and maintain the patient's plan of care.

Anxiety Disorders

Anxiety, the unpleasant feeling of fear and apprehension, is something that most people experience at one point or another in their lives. People have anxious feelings about taking tests, speaking in public, interacting with the opposite sex, making new friends and acquaintances, traveling to strange places, or personal circumstances. Common sources of anxiety are money, job-related, and family relationships. Anxiety of this nature is completely normal, as long it does not prevent people from living their lives, facing their minor fears or worries and moving forward.

Sometimes, though, some people find that they are paralyzed by their anxiety and cannot act. Instead of taking the actions they know they should, they retreat and avoid the situation entirely. This might not seem too harmful if it is a case of a person being afraid, for example, of tigers. As long as he or she doesn't live in an area populated by such animals, the situation might never present a problem. However, what happens if individuals have extreme anxiety in social situations to the point that they avoid interacting with others entirely? Or, if people are so afraid of germs that they cannot stop compulsively cleaning themselves to the point that they are unable to engage in normal activities for fear of contamination? It is at this point that individuals must seek professional help in order to conquer their fears so that they can live normal, full lives.

Chronic anxiety can interfere with an individual's ability to lead a normal life. Mental health professionals consider people who suffer from continued anxiety as having anxiety disorders. The physical symptoms of anxiety may include nervousness, fear, shortness of breath, dizziness, rapid heart rate, muscle tension, a "knot" in the stomach, sweating, or elevated blood pressure. If the anxiety is severe and long lasting, more serious problems may develop. People suffering from anxiety over an extended period may have headaches, ulcers, irritable bowel syndrome, trouble sleeping, and depression. Because anxiety tends to create various other emotional and physical symptoms, a "snowball" effect can occur in which these problems produce even more anxiety.

Interestingly, worry and negative thinking, considered common symptoms of anxiety, may also trigger it. Persons who have certain kinds of thinking—unrealistic and overly pessimistic—are at greater risk for anxiety disorders

Anxiety disorders—separation anxiety disorder, generalized anxiety disorder (GAD), social phobia, and obsessive-compulsive disorder—are the mental disorders that are most common among children and adolescents. Separation anxiety is normal among infants, toddlers, and very young children. For example, nearly every child experiences at least a momentary pang of separation anxiety on the first day of preschool or kindergarten. When this condition occurs in older children or adolescents and it is severe enough to impair social, academic, or job functioning for at least one month it is considered separation anxiety disorder. The risk factors associated with social anxiety disorder include stress such as the illness or death of a family member, geographic relocation, and physical or sexual assault.

Children with separation anxiety may be "clingy," and often they fear that accidents or natural disasters will forever separate them from their parents. Since they fear being apart from their parents they may resist going to school or going anywhere without a parent. Separation anxiety can produce physical symptoms such to dizziness, nausea, or rapid heart rate and is often associated with symptoms of depression. Young children may have difficulties falling asleep alone in their rooms and may have nightmares.

Children suffering from social anxiety disorder (also known as social phobia) are overly worried about being embarrassed in social situations. Although the degree to which social anxiety disorders harm children and teens varies, many are unable to speak in class, enter into conversation with peers, or eat, drink, or write in public. The anxiety produces physical symptoms such as blushing, sweating, and diarrhea. Young children may not be able to verbally express their fears, but may cry, cling, or avoid contact with others. Reluctant to attend school and unable to socialize with peers, children with social anxiety disorder may suffer from low self-esteem, viewing themselves as academic and social "failures." The disorder affects more girls than boys, and while it may become less severe or completely resolve over time, most sufferers are affected to some degree throughout their lives.

Phobias Phobias are defined as unreasonable fears of particular situations or objects. The most common of the many varieties of phobias are specific phobias. Bees, snakes, rodents, heights, closed spaces, odors, blood, injections, and thunderstorms are examples of common fears in specific phobias. Specific phobias, especially animal phobias, are common in children, but they can occur at any age. About 8% of American adults suffer from specific phobias. Most people with phobias understand that their fears are unreasonable, but that awareness does not make them feel any less anxious.

Specific phobias, such as a fear of heights, usually do not interfere with daily life or cause as much distress as more severe forms, such as agoraphobia (the fear of crowds and open spaces). This is a phobia that can impair a person's ability to connect with others, to attend school, and to hold a job. People with severe agoraphobia not only avoid crowds and busy places but also may refuse to leave their homes entirely.

Agoraphobia usually develops slowly, following a first, unexpected panic attack. For example, on an ordinary day, while shopping, driving to work, or doing errands, the person is suddenly struck by a wave of terror and symptoms such as trembling, a pounding heart, sweating, and difficulty breathing normally. The person desperately seeks safety, reassurance from friends and family, or a physician. The panic subsides, and all is well—until another panic attack occurs. Agoraphobia usually

What are You Afraid Of?

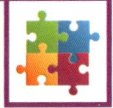

For every fear, it seems there is a phobia. Listed below are just some phobias, from the common to the plain weird.

- Ailurophobia (fear of cats)
- Bibliophobia (fear of books)
- Coulrophobia (fear of clowns)
- Didaskaleinophobia (fear of going to school)
- Entomophobia (fear of insects)
- Glossophobia (fear of speaking)
- Heliophobia (fear of the sun)
- Ichthyophobia (fear of fish)
- Lachanophobia (fear of vegetables)
- Myctophobia (fear of darkness)
- Nosocomephobia (fear of hospitals)
- Ophidiaphobia (fear of snakes)
- Pantophobia (fear of everything)
- Rupophobia (fear of dirt)
- Sophophobia (fear of learning)
- Triskadekaphobia (fear of the number 13)
- Urophobia (fear of urine or urinating)
- Xenophobia (fear of strangers or foreigners)
- Zoophobia (fear of animals)

begins during the late teens or twenties, and about 5% of the adult population suffers from agoraphobia. Women tend to be affected two times more often than are men. People suffering from severe specific phobias like agoraphobia may rearrange their lives drastically to avoid the situations they fear will trigger panic attacks.

Treatments. Treatments for phobias usually involve confronting the fear in some way. Behavioral therapists may use a variety of techniques that involve visualization or actual contact with the object or situation around which the phobia centers. The thinking behind this, for certain schools of therapies, is that it will desensitize the phobic to the phobia. For example, flooding, a behavioral technique, involves exposing a phobic person to the cause of the phobia in an extreme way; however, this

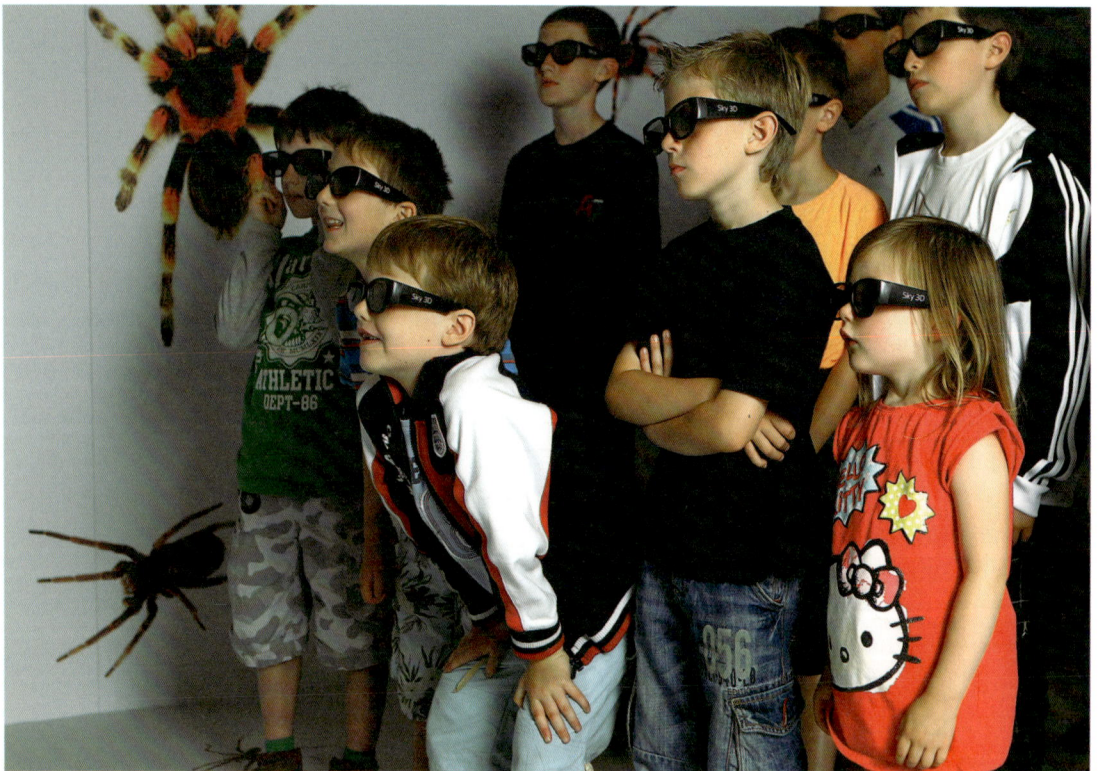

Kids view the launch of an arachnophobia therapy clinic. Arachnophobes will be shown 3D TV footage of domestic, wild, and dangerous spiders to help them overcome their fears of these eight-legged creatures in the ultimate immersion therapy.
© GETTY IMAGES.

can cause the phobic serious initial discomfort, at the very least, and many therapists shy away from therapies that could potentially traumatize a patient. A gentler kind of behavior modification known as *systematic desensitization* has been used to treat persons with phobias such as fear of flying in airplanes, fear of riding in elevators, and fears of spiders, snakes, and insects. This therapy involves learning to relax rather than feeling anxious or fearful in the face of progressively more threatening situations until exposure to the previously feared act or object no longer triggers anxiety.

Operant conditioning is also used to help people cope with phobias. Cognitive therapists will work with people with phobias using cognitive therapies alone (without some type of exposure to the source of the phobia), but this is usually effective only in the case of social phobias. Furthermore, people with social phobias have responded well to behavioral techniques that involve acquiring better social skills so that they feel more comfortable in social situations.

Panic Attacks and Panic Disorder A panic attack can accompany several different anxiety disorders, so in and of itself, a panic attack is not a separate disorder. Essentially, a panic attack is a short period involving intense feelings of fear or discomfort along with several telltale symptoms. These symptoms include an irregular or accelerated heart rate or a pounding of the heart; sweating, discomfort, or pain in the chest; a feeling of choking or not being able to breathe properly; trembling, feelings of detachment, of things being "unreal," and/or of impending doom. People experiencing panic attacks have described feeling as though they would lose control completely or were about to have a heart attack or stroke.

Panic attacks may be caused by certain situations, such as being in a strange place, but they can happen when people are relaxing or sleeping. If panic attacks continue to occur when there is no apparent stressor (stress-inducing event), a person might be diagnosed with panic disorder. Extremely high levels of anxiety may produce panic attacks that are both unexpected and seemingly without cause. In one type of panic attack, called "unexpected," the sufferer is unable to predict when an attack will occur. Other types of panic attacks are linked to a particular location, circumstance, or event and are called "situationally bound" or "situationally predisposed" panic attacks. These panic episodes can last as long as 30 minutes and are marked by an overwhelming sense of impending doom while the person's heart races and breathing quickens to the point of gasping for air. Sweating, nausea, weakness, dizziness, terror, and feelings of unreality are also typical.

Repeated panic attacks may be termed a panic disorder, however panic attacks do not necessarily indicate a mental disorder—as much as 10% of people with no other problems experience a single panic attack each year. According to the American Psychiatric Association, panic disorder occurs twice as often among women than men, and most sufferers begin to experience attacks between the ages of 15 and 19. Research has revealed that people who experience panic attacks tend to suppress their emotions. Some mental health professionals think that this tendency to crush and control feelings leads to an emotional buildup for which a panic attack is a form of release. Interestingly, most persons who suffer from panic attacks do not experience anxiety between attacks.

Panic disorder is a common ailment, affecting 2% of men and 5% of women. The disorder may be inherited: some researchers believe that panic attacks, like other mental disorders, may occur more frequently among persons with a specific genetic mutation. Other experts believe that panic disorders and phobias such as agoraphobia are solely psychological in origin. Furthermore, one set of researchers has even suggested that the agoraphobia that so often coexists with panic disorders isn't really a fear of public places but rather a fear of losing control and having a panic attack in a public place.

Certain drugs, such as antidepressants, have been used to treat people with panic disorder and agoraphobia with some success; however, the drugs are merely a temporary measure as symptoms return when people stop taking the drugs. Cognitive behavioral therapy helps many people lessen the severity of the disorder.

Obsessive-Compulsive Disorder People with obsessive-compulsive disorder (OCD) cannot control their thoughts or behaviors. OCD is an anxiety disorder marked by unwanted, often unpleasant recurring thoughts (obsessions) and repetitive, often mechanical behaviors (compulsions). The repetitive behaviors—such as continually checking to be certain windows and doors are locked or repeated hand washing—are intended to drive out the obsessive thoughts that trigger them, for example, that an intruder will enter the house through an unlocked door or window or that disease will be prevented by hand washing. Persons suffering from OCD may fear causing harm to others, fear making mistakes, and/or fear behaving in a socially unacceptable manner. Many also feel a tremendous need for symmetry and precision, creating systems to organize their possessions and experiencing severe distress when these systems are disturbed or disrupted. The vicious cycle of obsessions and compulsions only serves to increase anxiety. OCD can become the center of sufferers' lives and prevent them from doing the things they would like to do, at least in part because compulsive behaviors take up an inordinate amount of time.

While nearly everyone has some behavioral quirks like cracking knuckles or strong preferences such as wanting books on a shelf lined up in size order, obsessions and compulsions are different in that they prevent people from living normal lives. Examples of obsessions may include fear about becoming "contaminated" with germs, which causes the person with OCD to avoid shaking hands with others; or counting the words and lines on each page the person with OCD reads; or being convinced that he has left his front door unlocked. The compulsions accompanying these obsessions can include things such as repeatedly using hand sanitizer for fear of germs, or checking repeatedly (sometimes a certain number—for instance, three times) to see if they have indeed locked the front door. Unlike preferences, a compulsion is something that is viewed as not being part of someone's personality but rather irrational behavior that a person is unable to stop. OCD can separate people from others, because it leaves affected individuals unable to participate

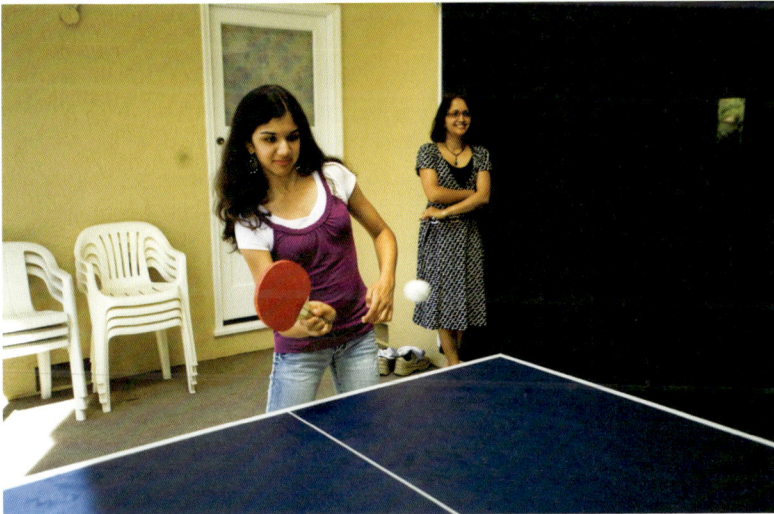

Nikita Desai plays table tennis at her home in as her mother watches. With treatment, Desai overcame OCD and started a Web site to help other teens with OCD, finding an expert to give advice to those using the site. The first symptoms of OCD often begin during childhood or adolescence. Desai wanted other kids with OCD to know they are not alone, and that OCD is a treatable disorder. © PAUL KITAGAKI/ SACRAMENTO BEE/MCT VIA GETTY IMAGES.

in everyday activities because their obsessions and compulsions prevent them from doing so.

Causes. OCD sometimes runs in families, which suggests that the tendency to develop it may be inherited. Researchers think that that a genetic defect may contribute to its development by changing levels of some chemicals, particularly serotonin, in the brain. There can also be organic (relating to the body) causes for OCD, such as head injuries and brain tumors as well as chemical imbalances in the brain. Behavioral and cognitive therapists believe that the behaviors and thinking related to OCD are learned and reinforced. For example, a person may have the irrational belief that she has not locked her door; by going back to check whether or not it is indeed locked, she is able to relieve the stress that is related to her worries. Some therapists also think that much of the problem stems from the fact that people suffering from OCD simply cannot remember whether or not they did something.

Treatments. Treating OCD is not an easy task, however cognitive behavior therapy is useful for treating OCD. It teaches people different ways of thinking, behaving, and reacting to situations that help them feel less anxious or fearful, which in turn reduces obsessive thoughts and compulsive behaviors. Another successful therapy, called exposure and response prevention, involves placing a person in a situation that usually triggers his anxiety, but not allowing the patient to engage in the compulsive behavior that would be his or her typical response. OCD patients learn new ways to manage their obsessive thoughts without resorting to compulsive behaviors, and over time the stress from not performing the compulsive behavior lessens to the point where the person no longer feels compelled to do it.

Prescription drugs, especially antidepressants, have also proven successful in reducing obsessive thoughts and compulsive behaviors; this approach will not necessarily resolve the problem entirely but may help enable people to live normal lives while working through the issues in therapy.

Post-Traumatic Stress Disorder Every day, people experience traumatic events, anything from having a car accident to being robbed or sexually assaulted or even witnessing such an event happening to someone else. While people may survive these events (which involve intense fear and a feeling of helplessness), and their physical injuries and wounds may heal, they may still carry emotional scars.

When an individual experiences emotional aftereffects from a traumatic event days, months, or even years after the actual event, this is known as post-traumatic stress disorder, or PTSD (the prefix "post" means after or later). Many of these people, much later, will relive the event, become extremely upset and/or have nightmares about the event. They may also try to avoid people, places, and things that remind them of the trauma. Because PTSD is an anxiety disorder, they may also be plagued by sleep problems, have difficulty concentrating, and startle easily and dramatically. People with PTSD may feel frightened even when they are not in danger.

PTSD usually receives a great deal of attention in the media when veterans return home from war. Today, many veterans who served in Afghanistan and Iraq suffer from and are being treated for PTSD. Reports of the effects of PTSD on people's lives were more frequent in the years following the Vietnam War (1954–75), as they had been after World Wars I (1914–17) and II (1939–45), the Korean Conflict (1950–53) and, in fact, even after earlier conflicts such as the American Civil War (1861–65), because of the emotional scars that those who had served in a war often seemed to display. In fact, PTSD was originally called "shell shock" (in reference to the ammunition used during times of war). It is now known that people who have witnessed or participated in any type of traumatic event—such as an earthquake, or being involved in the search-and-rescue or recovery missions for victims of plane crashes in which hundreds of people perish—are now known to be potential sufferers from PTSD. What is not yet known is why PTSD affects only certain people and not everyone who experienced the same or a similar devastating event.

Children and teens also can and do suffer from PTSD when they have seen or been involved in violent events or disasters, but their symptoms are different from those of adults. Very young children may backslide in behavior. For example, children already toilet-trained they may begin to wet the bed or may start to use baby talk again. Others may withdraw and become especially clingy, refusing to go anywhere without a parent. Other children will act out the scary event while they are playing, reliving their fears. Teens may suffer from guilt and anxiety and may think or talk about getting even or seeking revenge.

Treatments. Great strides have been made in treating PTSD through the use of psychotherapy and medication. Some people with

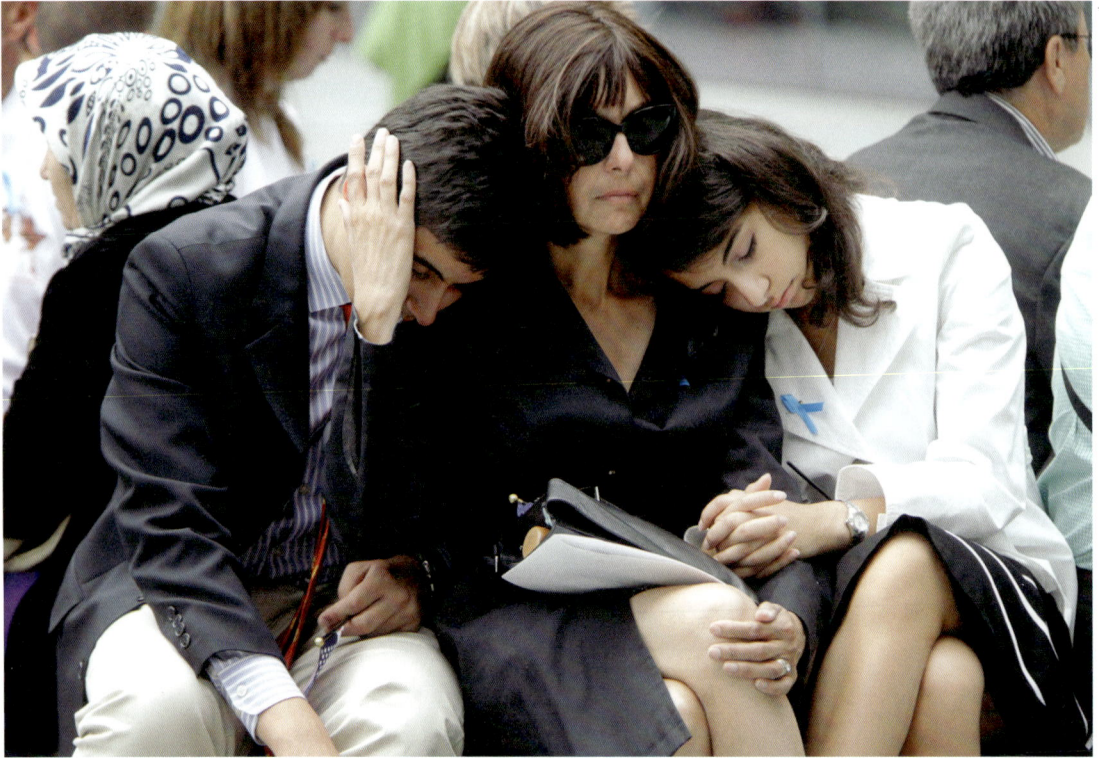

A woman comforts her children while visiting the National 9/11 Memorial during the 10th anniversary ceremonies of the September 11, 2001, terrorist attacks at the World Trade Center site in New York City. Many people who witnessed the attacks or had loved ones killed at the World Trade Center and the Pentagon that day experienced traumatic stress, and some still suffer from post traumatic stress disorder years later. © SETH WENIG/GETTY IMAGES.

PTSD benefit from cognitive behavioral therapy in individual sessions or group therapy. Talking in a group with others who have experienced similar events and have suffered from them continuously can be very helpful, because patients may feel that they are not alone in their feelings and that others understand the intensity of their traumatic experience. Most therapies, individual or group, usually involve dealing with or confronting the traumatic event in some way.

There is some evidence that PTSD can be prevented. People who live through traumatic events are encouraged to seek at least brief therapy to ensure that PTSD won't develop years later. Talk therapy helps people change how they react to their fear, guilt and shame after a traumatic event. They learn to make sense of bad memories, face and control their fear, and reduce their anxiety. They learn to relax, eat a healthful diet, exercise, and get enough sleep. Family and friends can help by listening and offering support, understanding and encouragement.

Other Types of Mental Disorders

There are other mental or psychological disorders that afflict millions of people each day. These can range from disorders most often appearing in old age, such as Alzheimer disease, to gender-identity disorders, in which people wish to be, or feel as though they are, members of the opposite sex. Eating disorders are also an increasingly common mental illness.

Somatoform Disorder Sometimes people complain of pain or discomfort that lingers but when they seek medical treatment, doctors can find no physical cause for the symptoms. When this persists, and the pain and discomfort prevent a person from participating in day-to-day life, a mental health professional may diagnose that person with pain disorder, which is just one of several somatoform disorders. Somatoform disorders are psychological disorders that manifest themselves physically without the presence of a true physical ailment. People suffering from them have physical complaints that may appear to result from medical problems but cannot be explained by a physical disease, substance abuse, or by another mental disorder.

Somatoform disorders can include conversion disorders, which can result in sudden loss of vision (once called hysterical blindness) or paralysis. People have also been known to lose their senses of hearing and smell as well. Another somatoform disorder is body dysmorphic disorder (BDD), which some people call "imagined ugliness." While many people would like to change something about themselves (such as being more muscular, having smaller ears, having straight or curly hair, being taller, shorter, or thinner), people with BDD grossly exaggerate what they perceive to be flaws in their appearance and spend hours obsessing about these so-called flaws. Some BDD sufferers even take measures to act upon their impulses by picking at their skin (if they think they have too many blemishes) or getting plastic surgery unnecessarily. Treatment of BDD may include medication and cognitive behavioral therapy.

As with many other mental disorders, there is no single theory that can account for why certain people develop somatoform disorders while

Baron Von Munchausen and Mental Illness

Baron Von Munchausen was an 18th-century German huntsman and soldier known for telling greatly exaggerated tales about his adventures and exploits. Because of his reputation and the publication of tales based on his anecdotes (written by Rudolph Erich Raspe), the name Munchausen is now associated with exaggeration. So it came to be that when people faked or dramatically exaggerated symptoms of illnesses, the disorder was named Munchausen syndrome. In addition, when a parent or guardian faked the illnesses of a child, by lying about the child's medical history or current condition in order to make others believe the child was ill, this was called Munchausen-by-proxy syndrome.

Although Munchausen syndrome and Munchausen-by-proxy syndrome are still recognizable names, and still in use, the proper clinical term for these syndromes is factitious disorders. Factitious disorders are mental disorders in which patients intentionally behave

as though they are physically or mentally ill without obvious benefits. Factitious disorders are very different from malingering, which is defined as pretending to have an illness with a clear motive, such as financial gain. Factitious disorders go beyond fibbing; they are serious psychological disorders, and have consequences that affect others.

Factitious disorders can threaten the life of an otherwise healthy child, because the disturbed caretaker may even go so far as to injure the child or taint blood or urine specimens to sustain the illusion of illness. There is no single cause of factitious disorders. Some researchers think underlying personality disorders; child abuse; or the wish to deceive or test authority figures may contribute to the development of this disorder. Other experts point to a warped need for attention or to be cared for; incomplete recovery from a major personal loss or trauma; or the desire for an abnormally intense and dependent relationship with the child.

others do not. Oftentimes, a person will recover suddenly from the problem while others require therapy. As with other mental disorders, there is evidence that some combination of inherited traits may contribute to the risk for and development of somatoform disorders. Researchers believe some triggers may include: brain chemistry, particularly neurotransmitters, brain chemicals involved in regulating mood; pre-birth environmental exposures such as exposure to viruses, toxins, or alcohol in the womb; and life experiences such as extreme stress or physical or emotional abuse.

Dissociative Disorder When someone dissociates, it means that a certain behavior or part of the personality becomes removed from the rest of his or her consciousness. This can be something as harmless as losing track of time while reading a terrific book or becoming preoccupied while listening to a song on an iPod while walking and forgetting which route was taken upon arriving at a destination. However, dissociation can also be a very serious problem, and several disorders are attached to this phenomenon.

There are four major dissociative disorders—dissociative amnesia, dissociative fugue, dissociative identity disorder, and depersonalization disorder:

Dissociative Amnesia. Dissociative amnesia involves memory loss that is not caused by a medical condition. People with this disorder cannot remember personal information, such as where they have been, who they are, events or people in their lives, or entire recent conversations. Often this is prompted by a stressful event, such as abuse, trauma, or the death of a loved one.

Dissociative Fugue. Dissociative fugue (pronounced fyoog) is a particularly disturbing mental phenomenon as it involves one or more instances of a person leaving their normal, everyday life for a period of time while taking up a new life with no recollection of their former life. Like dissociative amnesia, fugues are often triggered by traumatic events and are often fueled by unfulfilled wishes. An individual in the midst of a fugue will often leave home, abandoning all aspects of his or her life, and assume a new identity in another place. A fugue can last hours or days or longer. When it ends, affected individuals may feel out of sorts but they generally have no memory of what happened during the fugue.

Dissociative Identity Disorder. Dissociative identity disorder, or DID (formerly known as multiple personality disorder, or MPD), involves an individual having two or more identities or personalities that are in control of the person's behaviors and thoughts at different times. Each identity has a different name, history, and unique characteristics, including apparent differences in voice, gender, mannerisms, and even such physical characteristics such as the need for glasses or use of a cane. People diagnosed with DID will often have a variety of personalities that are very different from one another and that may even be in opposition to one another. For example, one personality may be left-handed whereas the other(s) are right-handed. DID usually begins in childhood and is often the result of severe trauma or repressing (consciously rejecting, holding back, or suppressing) strong feelings and desires.

Depersonalization Disorder. This disorder is marked by a sudden sense of being outside of oneself, watching one's actions from a distance

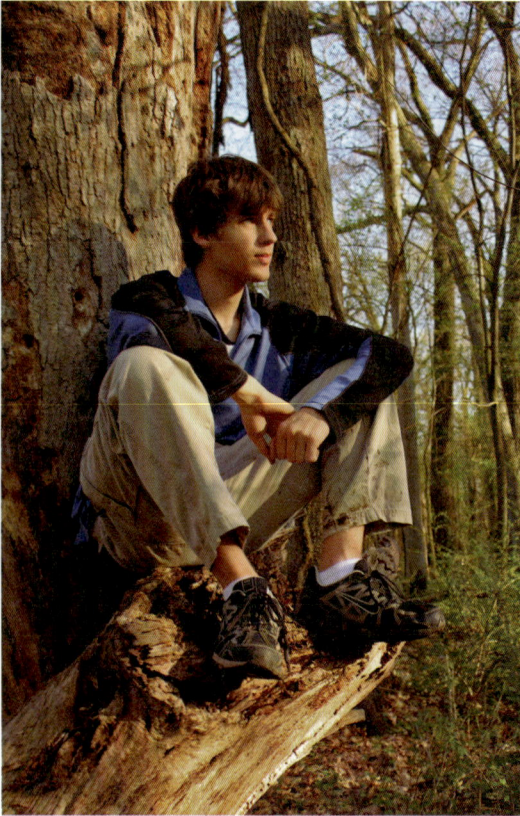

Though most people have moments in which they may lose track of time or forget what they are doing momentarily, those suffering with depersonalization disorder may have long periods in which they feel detached from their own bodies, thoughts, or emotions, which may lead to increasing feelings of dissociation from the rest of society and isolation. This, in turn leads to a cycle of increasing anxiety, which further exacerbates the problem.
© DOUBLE PHOTOGRAPHY/
SHUTTERSTOCK.COM.

as though watching a movie. The size and shape of objects or people may seem altered. Time may seem to slow down, and the world may seem unreal. These symptoms may last for only a few moments or may return periodically over time.

Because of the association of the concept of repression with dissociative disorders, psychoanalytic therapists seem to have had good success in treating these disorders. Hypnosis and art therapies also may be used by therapists to help uncover forgotten or repressed memories in order to get to the root causes of individuals' feelings of disconnection from themselves. Some people with these disorders also benefit from antidepressants or anti-anxiety medications to help control their symptoms.

Personality Disorders People have different personalities that are expressed as different behavioral and emotional traits. Many people, however, share a type of personality, which means they have certain tendencies. For example, someone who is very sensitive to criticism might have an avoidant personality type. This is perfectly acceptable unless that person's behavior is extreme, in which case it might present problems in personal relationships and the ability to function in society. If the person with this personality type avoids people in social and work-related situations because of fear of being criticized or rejected; shies away from getting close to other people for fear of being made fun of; has low self-esteem; and is painfully shy and standoffish, then he or she might have an avoidant personality disorder. In other words, the difference between a personality type and a personality disorder is that the disorder separates people from others and the separation can prevent them from being happy and successful.

People with personality disorders have unhealthy patterns of thinking and behaving, and these patterns may cause them to have serious problems in relationships, social interactions, work, and school. Symptoms of personality disorders include frequent and dramatic mood swings, troubled relationships, social isolation, angry and sometimes violent outbursts, trouble making and keeping friends, difficulty controlling one's impulses, the need for immediate gratification, and alcohol or substance abuse.

There is a wide range of personality disorders. There is the histrionic personality disorder, in which the affected individual is excessively emotional; needs to be the center of attention; behaves inappropriately (making sexual comments, for example); wears revealing clothes; is overly dramatic; is easily influenced by other people or events; and exaggerates how emotionally close he or she is actually is to another person.

Dependent personality disorder is marked by an overwhelming need for advice and reassurance from others; being unable to disagree with others for fear he or she will no longer be liked; having a lack of initiative and self-direction; and showing an unusual need for close relationships along with a fear of being alone.

Other personality disorders include the paranoid personality disorder, in which there is constant distrust and suspicion of other people and the affected individuals think others are "out to get them." People with paranoid personality disorder may be hostile or emotionally detached.

There is also the schizotypal personality disorder in which people are removed from social contact with others and have problems experiencing and expressing emotion. People with this disorder may have "magical thinking," the belief that they can influence others with their thoughts, and they may think that there are secret messages for them in public speeches, songs, or other media.

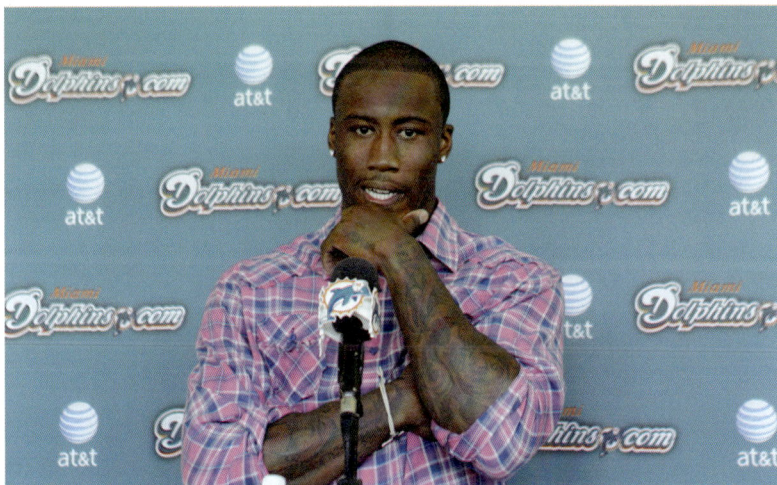

Miami Dolphins wide receiver Brandon Marshall (traded to the Chicago Bears in 2012) talks to reporters in 2011. Marshall was diagnosed with borderline personality disorder (BPD), sometimes characterized by unstable relationships, negative self-image, and fear of failure. Marshall's career has been successful, but marred by trouble off the field. He stated he would like to raise awareness of BPD.
© AP IMAGES/J PAT CARTER.

In borderline personality disorder people are unstable in their relationships with others, have poor self-image, unstable moods, and are very impulsive. They may fear being alone and are at risk for suicide attempts.

People with narcissistic personality disorder are overly conceited, have an abnormal need for admiration, and exhibit a lack of empathy for others—they do not recognize other people's emotions and feelings. People with this disorder crave power, success, and attention; tend to exaggerate their accomplishments; and seek praise and admiration.

Personality disorders are treated differently, depending on which type of disorder is present. Treatment may involve psychotherapy, medication, or even hospitalization. The success of therapy depends on the active participation of the patient and his or her willingness to follow the prescribed treatment plan. The challenge in treating personality disorders is that patients with these disorders tend to act in ways that affect treatment and their personal safety. For instance, people with severe personality disorders often engage in high-risk behavior, such as excessive drinking or taking illegal drugs. Furthermore, they are less likely to take medications prescribed to them in the proper manner, and have a hard time taking responsibility for their behavior or trusting their mental health care providers.

For More Information

BOOKS

Cooper, Barbara, and Nancy Widdows. *The Social Success Workbook for Teens: Skill-Building Activities for Teens with Nonverbal Learning Disorder, Asperger's Disorder, and Other Social-Skill Problems.* Oakland, CA: Instant Help, 2008.

Dawson, Peg, and Richard Guare *Smart but Scattered: The Revolutionary "Executive Skills" Approach to Helping Kids Reach Their Potential.* New York: Guilford Press, 2013.

Ford, Emily, Michael Liebowitz, and Linda Wasmer Andrews *What You Must Think of Me: A Firsthand Account of One Teenager's Experience with Social Anxiety Disorder.* New York: New York: Oxford University Press, 2007.

Hutchins Paquette, Penny, and Cheryl Gerson Tuttle. *Learning Disabilities: The Ultimate Teen Guide (It Happened to Me).* Lanham, MD: Scarecrow Press, 2006.

Jamieson, Patrick E., and Moira A. Rynn *Mind Race: A Firsthand Account of One Teenager's Experience with Bipolar Disorder.* New York: Oxford University Press, 2006.

Schab, Lisa M. *Beyond the Blues: A Workbook to Help Teens Overcome Depression.* Oakland, CA: Instant Help Books, 2008.

Schab, Lisa M. *The Anxiety Workbook for Teens.* Oakland, CA: Instant Help Books, 2008.

Van Dijk, Sheri. *Don't Let Your Emotions Run Your Life for Teens: Dialectical Behavior Therapy Skills for Helping You Manage Mood Swings, Control Angry Outbursts, and Get Along with Others.* Oakland, CA: Instant Help Books, 2011.

WEB SITES

American Psychiatric Association. http://www.psych.org (accessed December 7, 2012).

American Psychological Association. http://www.apa.org/ (accessed December 7, 2012).

"Child and Adolescent Mental Health." *National Institute of Mental Health (NIMH).* http://www.nimh.nih.gov (accessed December 7, 2012).

National Alliance on Mental Illness. http://www.nami.org (accessed December 7, 2012).

National Institute of Mental Health (NIMH). http://www.nimh.nih.gov (accessed December 7, 2012).

The Nemours Foundation. "TeensHealth: Mind." *KidsHealth.org.* http://kidshealth.org/teen/your_mind/ (accessed December 7, 2012).

Teen Mental Health. http://www.teenmentalhealth.org/ (accessed December 7, 2012).

"Teen Mental Health." *Medline Plus.* http://www.nlm.nih.gov/medlineplus/teenmentalhealth.html (accessed December 7, 2012).

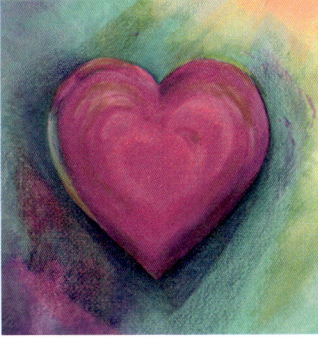

Behaviors, Habits, Addictions, and Eating Disorders

Introduction **531**

Addiction **531**

Substance Abuse **535**

Depressants **539**

Stimulants **543**

Hallucinogens **547**

Inhalants **550**

Alcohol and Alcoholism **550**

Nicotine **553**

Caffeine **554**

Treatment for Addiction **554**

Compulsive Behaviors **558**

Eating Disorders **563**

Causes of Eating Disorders **567**

The Physical and Psychological Consequences of Eating Disorders **571**

Eating Disorders and Other Destructive Behaviors **576**

Eating Disorders and Sexuality **576**

Treatment and Recovery from Eating Disorders **577**

Preventing Eating Disorders **579**

Developing a Positive Body Image **580**

For More Information **582**

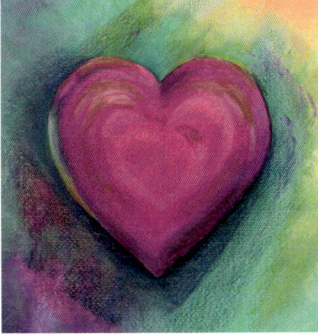

Behaviors, Habits, Addictions, and Eating Disorders

A habit is a way of behaving that is repeated so often it no longer involves conscious thought. Examples of habits are brushing one's teeth every morning before school and evening before bed, or walking the dog every morning before school or work. These habits typically are considered "good" habits to have because they are of benefit to the person performing them. Other habits, such as stealing an item from a department store at each visit to the store or drinking alcohol to excess frequently at a friend's house, would typically be considered "bad" habits because they may bring harm to the person performing them.

Another definition of habit is an addiction. Both good and bad habits can be addictive in nature. When someone eats a healthful cereal with fruit for breakfast every morning, that person has established a good habit because it is important to eat a nutritious breakfast every day. If, though, the person became so dependent on eating a particular brand of cereal every morning that his mood changed for the worse if he was unable to eat the cereal one morning, his habit would be more serious. One could argue that he was addicted to the cereal. Of course one can't become physically addicted to a brand of cereal the way one can become physically addicted, for example, to the nicotine in cigarettes, but this does serve as an example of how a habit can sometimes turn into an addictive behavior.

This chapter focuses on several types of negative habits and behaviors and ways to treat them. From substance abuse and eating disorders to Internet addiction and gambling, these habits can pose potentially life-threatening risks.

Addiction

Addiction is a physical or mental need for a substance or activity. It is most commonly defined as dependence on harmful, habit-forming drugs. When most people think of the word addiction, they conjure

Words to Know

Addiction: The physical or mental need for a substance or the state of needing to compulsively repeat a behavior.

Adrenaline: Also known as epinephrine, adrenaline is a hormone that is released during times of stress that causes the heart rate to increase and strengthens the force of the heart's contraction. Secretion of adrenaline is part of the human "fight or flight" response to fear, panic, or perceived threat. Adrenaline also blocks the histamine response in an allergic reaction.

Altered consciousness: A state of awareness that is different from typical, waking consciousness; often induced with the use of drugs and alcohol.

Amenorrhea: The absence of menstrual cycles.

Anorexia nervosa: A term meaning "lack of appetite"; an eating disorder marked by a person's refusal or inability to maintain a healthy body weight resulting from restricting food intake or other means.

Benign: Harmless; also, non-cancerous.

Binge-eating disorder: An eating disorder that involves repetitive episodes of binge eating in a restricted period of time over several months.

Bingeing: When an individual eats an abnormally large amount of food in a particular period of time.

Body set-point theory: A theory of weight control that claims that the body will defend a certain weight regardless of factors such as calorie intake and exercise.

Bulimia nervosa: A term that means literally "ox hunger"; an eating disorder characterized by a repeated cycle of bingeing and purging.

Compulsive behavior: Behavior that is repeated over and over again, uncontrollably.

Crash: Coming down from being high on drugs or alcohol.

Cut: The habit of mixing illegal drugs with another substance to produce a greater quantity of that substance.

Delirium: Mental disturbance marked by confusion, disordered speech, and even hallucinations.

Depression: A disorder marked by intense and prolonged feelings of sadness, emptiness, hopelessness, and irritability, as well as a lack of pleasure in activities.

Detoxification: The process of freeing an individual of an intoxicating or addictive substance in the body or to free from dependence. Also, when doctors use medication to reduce or eliminate drugs or alcohol from a person's body.

Diuretic: A drug that increases the output of water from the body through urination.

Edema: Swelling.

Endorphin: Any of a group of natural proteins in the brain and nervous system that act as the body's natural pain relievers. Endorphins are released after exercise, causing people to feel better after exercise. Endorphins also affect emotions, helping people feel calm and content.

Enema: A process that expels waste from the body by injecting liquid into the anus.

Epidemiology: The study of disease in a population.

Euphoric: Having the feeling of well-being or elation.

Exercise addiction: Also known as compulsive exercise, a condition in which participation in exercise activities is taken to an extreme; people exercise to the detriment of all other things in their lives.

Genetic: Something present in the genes that is inherited from a person's biological parents.

Habit: A behavior or routine that is repeated.

Hallucination: The perception of seeing or hearing things when they aren't really present.

Hangover: The syndrome that occurs after being high on drugs or drinking alcohol, often including nausea, headache, dizziness, and fuzzy-mindedness.

Hypertension: High blood pressure.

Inhalants: Substances that people sniff to get high.

Kleptomania: Habitual stealing.

Lanugo: Fine hair that grows all over the body to keep it warm when the body lacks enough fat to accomplish this.

Laxatives: Medications that are given to treat constipation by inducing bowel movements. They may work by increasing the bulk of the stool, holding water within the stool, softening the stool, or stimulating the intestines to contract more vigorously.

Mantra: A phrase repeated during meditation to center the mind.

Meditation: A practice that helps one to center and focus the mind; sometimes used to help recovering addicts.

Obesity: The condition of being very overweight, marked by too much body fat.

Overdose: A dangerous, often deadly, reaction to taking too much of a certain drug.

Perception: One's consciousness and way of observing things.

Predisposition: To be susceptible to something.

Psychoactive: Something that affects brain function, mood, and behavior.

Psychological vulnerability: Used to describe people who may be at risk for drug addiction because of prior experiences or other influences.

Purging: When a person gets rid of the food that she has eaten by vomiting, taking an excessive amount of laxatives, diuretics, or enemas, or engaging in fasting and/or excessive exercise.

Pyromania: Habitual need to start fires.

Ritual: Observances or ceremonies that mark change, renewal, or other events.

Russell's sign: Calluses, cuts, and sores on the knuckles from repeated self-induced vomiting.

Self-medicate: When a person treats an ailment, mental or physical, with alcohol or drugs rather than seeing a physician or mental health professional.

Synthetic: Something that is human-made; not occurring in nature.

Tolerance: The build-up of resistance to the effects of a substance.

Withdrawal: The phase of removal of drugs or alcohol from the system of the user.

images of a world they expect never to know. They imagine emaciated heroin addicts in dark alleys or remember rock stars that died as a result of overdoses. Addiction doesn't always look as menacing as public-service announcements or after-school television programs depict it. In fact, many people come into contact with some kind of addiction every day or are addicted to some substance they might consider benign (harmless). While addiction is common, becoming addicted to a substance or an activity can have serious consequences. And it's not something that just happens to "other" people.

Many adults, and an increasing number of teenagers, drink coffee first thing every morning. In fact, many people feel that without their first cup, normal daily functioning would be impossible. This reflects the problem inherent to addiction—the need itself. The subject of the addiction may seem harmless or even healthy (such as exercise addiction), but too much of anything can be dangerous. Having a cup of coffee to start the day is not a problem; however, it is possible to become addicted to caffeine (the addictive substance in coffee). Although there is not much attention paid to caffeine as a drug of addiction because it doesn't have many of the health and social consequences associated with addiction to alcohol, prescription, and illegal drugs, it "hooks" people much the same way.

In the case of alcoholics (those addicted to alcohol), many feel that they must have a drink before they can socialize. Addictions of all types, whether they are to hard drugs, such as heroin, or everyday substances, such as caffeine or sugar, can disrupt people's lives and ruin their mental and physical well-being. Addiction to drugs and alcohol, because they are mind-altering substances, poses more of a direct threat to users than do substances that don't immediately change people's perceptions.

Dependence Addiction is dependence. Infants, for example, are dependent on their parents for sustenance and other basic needs, such as shelter. Addicted people are dependent on a substance to function normally and feel good. Addicts are scared of the consequences of separation from their substance of choice. Addicted people exist at many levels of functioning and degrees of healing. There are addicts in all walks of life, from physicians and attorneys to schoolteachers and actors. Some of these addicted people are able to perform their jobs without anyone else becoming aware of their problems. They are able to fool others into thinking they can function normally. But others are seriously harmed:

their addictions prevent them from holding onto jobs or even engaging in activities with family and friends.

To truly heal and recover from addiction, addicts need to admit to themselves that they need help. Recovery from addiction is a process that involves taking a good, hard look at one's self. Self-examination can be quite intimidating, and many people would rather avoid it and hide in drinking, drugging, or codependency (extreme emotional or psychological reliance on someone with an illness or addiction). Self-discovery not only means uncovering the positive attributes a person may be unaware of; but also means coming to terms with shortcomings, flaws, and inadequacies and learning to accept those qualities.

Learning about the different forms of addiction and tools for recovery and healing can help those suffering from it. These coping strategies can help friends and families of people with addictions, too.

Substance Abuse

Most people who use drugs are seeking an altered state of consciousness. The need to alter consciousness is not a new phenomenon. Historical evidence shows that people of all cultures and eras have experimented with mind-altering substances, both natural and synthetic (human-made or artificial). People who use drugs seek to make the world around them look and feel different. This might mean trying to make a bleak life seem better or simply more interesting.

Drugs often make people feel confident and powerful. That's why taking drugs is called "getting high." Drugs give users a false sense of power that, of course, recedes when the artificial high ends. Addiction occurs when a person compulsively attempts to continue that high by taking a drug over and over again.

People use drugs for many, many reasons. For example, adolescents have reported that they experimented with marijuana to enhance sexuality; to feel more confident; for pleasure and relaxation; to make themselves more comfortable in social situations; to understand themselves better; for acceptance by their peers or to achieve elevated social status; to defy authority; and to expand their minds.

There are many theories about why some people choose to use drugs when others do not. Initial experimentation and addiction are two very different behaviors, though. The reason many people continue to seek out drugs after their first use is, again, an attempt to reproduce the same pleasure and an altered state of consciousness initially achieved the first time a certain drug was used. The second time and each instance thereafter, a user is trying to recapture the intensity of that first experience. Ultimately, these feelings cannot be replicated, and this is when an addiction starts. Drug users in search of that elusive pleasure will continue to search for the feelings inspired by their first time, even if all the consecutive uses affect them adversely; this is particularly dangerous with crack cocaine. (Many drug experts suggest that the initial experience of using crack cocaine is so intense that it takes only one use to kick-start an addiction.) Furthermore, over time, addicts' bodies develop a tolerance for a drug, meaning they will eventually have to take more and more of their drug of choice each time they use in order to achieve the same high.

Addiction counselors and others who work with substance abusers consider drug use and abuse to be a self-destructive behavior. According to this model, the user may not be consciously aware of being deeply depressed and engaging in self-destructive activities. Psychoanalytic counselors also interpret drug abuse as a form of suicidal behavior. Proponents of psychoanalysis believe that an addict is usually unaware of his or her deep-rooted problems, and the addiction is a symptom of unreleased pain resulting from these buried problems.

Causes of Substance Abuse There isn't one single cause of drug addiction. This is one of the reasons drug addiction is very hard to treat. Years ago the term "addictive personality" became very popular in the media. Many in the drug and alcohol addiction counseling field consider this term misleading because it suggests that drug abusers are to blame for their illness because they have defective personalities. A better way to describe a person's predisposition to substance abuse might be psychological (mind-related) vulnerability. This means that the addict has or had some prior psychological factor that placed him or her at greater risk for substance abuse.

For example, people who have mood disorders may sometimes self-medicate (make themselves feel better or more in balance) by using prescription or illegal drugs. There are a number of personality traits that are thought to be shared by substance abusers. These traits include high emotionality; anxiety; immaturity in relationships; low frustration tolerance; inability to express anger; problems with authority; low self-esteem; perfectionism; compulsiveness; feelings of isolation; sex-role confusion; depression; hostility; and sexual immaturity. Stress is also

Lost to Drugs

Many actors and musicians have waged well-documented battles with addiction, whether it be to drugs or alcohol. Some have come out triumphant, such as Drew Barrymore, who battled alcoholism at a very young age, and Matthew Perry, who triumphed over an addiction to painkillers.

Unfortunately, though, many talented individuals have lost their lives to drugs. In the early 1970s, the world of rock-and-roll mourned the overdose deaths of three musical giants, Jimi Hendrix, Janis Joplin, and Jim Morrison. During the 1980s and 1990s, John Bonham, the drummer with Led Zeppelin, died after drinking too much alcohol; Shannon Hoon, lead singer of the rock group Blind Melon, and Hillel Slovak, the original guitarist of the Red Hot Chili Peppers, both died of heroin overdoses; Brent Mydland of the Grateful Dead and Aaron West Arkeen, who wrote songs for Guns N' Roses, both died as a result of a drug overdoses. Since 2000, the deaths of Allen Woody of the Allman Brothers, Zac Foley of EMF, Layne Staley and Mike Starr of Alice in Chains, Dee Dee Ramone of the Ramones, Paul Gray of Slipknot, Mikey Welsh of Weezer, John Entwistle of The Who, Howie Epstein of Tom Petty and the Heartbreakers, Gidget Gein of Marilyn Manson, Jay Bennett of Wilco, Ike Turner, Michael Jackson, Whitney Houston, and Amy Winehouse were all related to drug or alcohol use.

Hollywood has lost its share of beloved performers as well. Actress Judy Garland, who played Dorothy in *The Wizard of Oz*, died in 1969 of an overdose from drugs, as did actor River Phoenix in 1995 at the age of 23. In 1997, comedian Chris Farley, age 33, died of a drug overdose as well, following in the footsteps of his own idol, actor/comedian John Belushi, who overdosed in 1982 also at the age of 33. More recent deaths attributed to drug use include actress Anna Nicole Smith in 2007, actors Heath Ledger and Brad Renfro in 2008, Brittany Murphy in 2009, and actor Corey Haim in 2010.

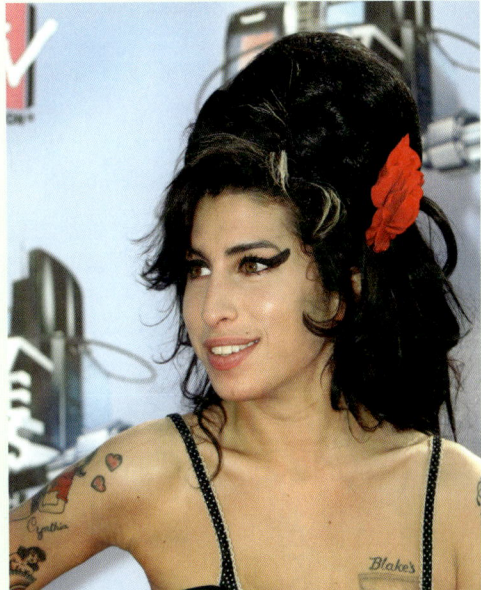

Amy Winehouse was a British singer and songwriter who won numerous awards, including five Grammies in 2008. She struggled for years with addictions to alcohol and drugs, including crack cocaine, heroin, and ecstasy. While trying to wean herself off of drugs, she began binge drinking. She died on July 23, 2011, at the age of 27, from alcohol poisoning. © ALLSTAR PICTURE LIBRARY/ALAMY.

thought to be a factor contributing to substance abuse. This is not referring to run-of-the-mill, everyday stress from work or school, but the kind of stress that is the result of traumatic experiences, such as the sudden loss of a loved one. Stress in early childhood, such as having been sexually or physically abused, can also lead to substance abuse.

A sense of self is one of the most important factors in the potential for drug addiction. People with a strong sense of self appreciate their individuality and are aware of their talents and place in the world. They are able to begin, develop, and complete projects and to coexist comfortably in different types of relationships. People with a weak sense of self are more likely to seek out alcohol and drugs as way to boost their sense of self, but it quickly vanishes once the drug wears off.

According to addiction counselors and researchers, preventing substance abuse in young people is more about giving them good reasons to live and helping them to foster a strong sense of self rather than keeping them away from the dangerous and enticing world of drugs.

Families and Drug Abuse A family history of substance abuse is another powerful risk factor. Because substance abuse tends to run in families, much research has focused on pinpointing the genetic predisposition to substance abuse. Twin studies have found that the rates of use, abuse, or dependence on alcohol and drugs are higher for identical twins that have exactly the same genetic makeup than for fraternal twins that only share some genes. Other research found that genetic influences are stronger for abuse of some drugs than for others, and that abusing any category of drugs—such as sedatives, stimulants, opiates, or heroin—was associated with a greater likelihood of abusing every other category of drugs. Also, each category of drug had unique genetic influences, and heroin was the drug with the greatest genetic influence for abuse.

Family and social environmental factors also influence whether an individual begins using drugs. A poorly functioning family system may contribute to the development of an addiction just as powerfully as a genetic predisposition.

Adolescence is a time of change and risk. Because teens are just beginning to develop their fragile sense of self, they are more prone to fall victim to substance abuse. This vulnerability is heightened because teens are exploring identity, social skills, and independence. Peer pressure, the need to fit in and be liked, often causes teens to experiment with alcohol and drugs. If a teen is at a party and everyone around is partying, one

A recent study found that nonmedical use of prescription pain medication, especially among adolescents, has increased in recent years. Teenage girls ages 15–19 are nearly twice as likely to abuse prescription pain medications as any other age group, and teen boys are 87% more likely to abuse pain medications than any other age group. The prescription pain medication teens abuse often comes from the medicine cabinets of parents, other family members, or friends.

might feel compelled to take a drink or smoke cigarettes or marijuana. Usually these situations do not occur as they do in the movies, where other kids actually pressure their peers; rather, peer pressure tends to work in more subtle ways. If a teen is feeling left out and alone at a party, he or she might believe that joining others smoking marijuana will help to gain acceptance into a group of friends. This is a reflection of teens' needs to feel as though they are part of a group—that they belong.

A teen feeling like the odd one out might even turn to doing drugs in private as a way to escape the frustration or pain of loneliness. Since drugs and alcohol are often easily available to teens, and avoiding contact with them is often difficult, many teens will have encounters with substance abuse either with themselves or people they know. Willpower and a strong sense of self seem to be qualities that keep people from giving in to substance use, abuse, and addiction.

Drugs: In the Medicine Cabinet and on the Street

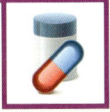

Psychoactive drugs are those that affect brain functions, mood, and behavior. Non-psychoactive drugs are substances that in normal doses do not directly affect the brain. There are several different categories of psychoactive drugs. There are over-the-counter and prescription drugs that fall into the category of psychoactive agents, as well as illegal or street drugs such as marijuana, heroin, or cocaine. All can carry the risk of addiction. It's important to remember that the effects of any drug depend on several variables. They are the amount taken at one time, the user's past drug experience, the method of administration (how the drug is taken—inhaled, smoked, swallowed), and the circumstances under which the drug is taken.

Depressants

Depressants are the family of substances that slow down, or depress, bodily functions. They tend to make the user sleepy or sluggish. The following drugs are depressants.

Narcotics Narcotics include opioids, the class of drugs derived from the poppy plant and the synthetic or semi-synthetic compounds that mimic opiates. Opiates, drugs derived from the natural alkaloids of the poppy plant, have been used for thousands of years in Asia both for pleasure and medicinal uses. Natural opiates include morphine, codeine, and heroin. Synthetic or semi-synthetic opioids include fentanyl, oxycodone, and meperidine. They cause a wide variety of effects and side effects, such as pain relief, euphoria, respiratory depression, drowsiness, constriction of the pupils, nausea and vomiting, itching, and constipation. Narcotics tend to be easily addictive when used regularly because of their quick and powerful effects.

Sharing Needles

Injecting drugs (using drugs by shooting them directly in to a vein with a needle) carries an even more deadly threat to the body than administering them in other ways, such as smoking or snorting. Heroin addicts, and others, who shoot drugs and share needles are in one of the highest risk groups for infection with hepatitis and human immunodeficiency virus (HIV), which can lead to acquired immunodeficiency syndrome (AIDS). HIV and hepatitis are transferred from person to person via bodily fluids. If the blood from an infected person is transferred to another person via a used needle, that person is at great risk of contracting these life-threatening diseases.

Narcotics can be ingested, injected, snorted, or smoked. When opioids are smoked, it takes just five seconds for the drug to reach the brain. If a person addicted to narcotics is without that drug for even four to six hours after the narcotic use stops, he or she can feel the beginnings of withdrawal.

Tolerance to Narcotics. Tolerance (the ability to resist the effects of something) develops quickly with the use of narcotics. Users must take more and more of the drug to get the desired effect. This can lead to overdose. Detoxification (cleansing the body of a toxic substance) is necessary for the body to recover. In order to detoxify and cleanse the body of the drug, withdrawal must occur. Withdrawal is the experience of ridding the body of the substance to which it has become accustomed. Withdrawal from opioids can cause a wide range of symptoms including: appetite suppression; nausea and vomiting; dilated pupils; gooseflesh; restlessness; intestinal spasm; abdominal pain; muscle spasms; kicking movements (the reason for the expression, "kicking the habit"); diarrhea; increased heart rate and blood pressure; chills, hot flashes, and sweating; irritability; insomnia; violent yawning; severe sneezing and runny nose; crying and tearing; nasal inflammation; and depressive moods and tremors.

Without treatment, withdrawal symptoms may last from seven to 10 days. Most opioid withdrawal symptoms are very uncomfortable but are not life threatening. When withdrawal occurs under medical supervision, medications may be given to reduce symptoms such as anxiety, agitation, muscle aches, sweating, runny nose, cramping, vomiting, and diarrhea.

Anti-Anxiety Drugs and Sleep Aids Benzodiazepines and barbiturates are in the sedative-hypnotic class of drugs and are usually prescribed by doctors for anxiety disorders or to induce sleep; benzodiazepines, such as Valium (diazepam), Ativan (lorazepam), Klonopin (clonazepam), and Xanax (alprazolam) are the most commonly prescribed anti-anxiety drugs. These drugs also may be prescribed as relaxants or sleep aids. Long-term use of benzodiazepines can be addicting, and they are often taken in combination with other drugs by patients with addiction disorders. (It is important to remember that even if a doctor prescribes a drug for someone, that person can abuse the drug and become addicted to it.) Commonly prescribed barbiturates include amobarbital, pentobarbital, butabarbital, phenobarbital, secobarbital, and methylphenobarbital.

Anti-anxiety drugs and sleep aids are taken orally, in pill form. They cause drowsiness, relaxation, and a sense of well-being. Effects are similar to those of alcohol. When used over any extended period of time, barbiturates can cause extreme physical and psychological dependence. Tolerance to the euphoric effects occur quickly, so more and more must be used to develop the desired effect. Withdrawal may cause dizziness, weakness, sleeplessness, anxiety, tremors, nausea, vomiting, delirium, delusions, and hallucinations.

Overdose is common with these types of drugs. In fact, they are often the drugs of choice for people attempting to commit suicide. Symptoms of overdose are severe mood alteration; confusion and disorientation; slurred speech; impaired motor coordination; involuntary rapid eye movement from side to side; dilated pupils; and respiratory depression.

There are other drugs with barbiturate-like effects that are not classified as barbiturates, such as methaqualone, better known by the trade name, Quaaludes, or the street name ludes. Quaaludes were thought to be a nonaddictive alternative to barbiturates when they were introduced in the 1960s. They turned out to have high abuse potential. They're very popular with college and high school students and have been illegal since 1984. They are often mixed with alcohol, creating a deadly combination. They produce sedation and sleep. Methoqualone may cause headaches, hangovers, fatigue, dizziness, drowsiness, menstrual disturbances, dry mouth, nosebleeds, diarrhea, skin eruptions, numbness, and pain in the arms and legs. Eight to 20 grams can produce severe toxicity, coma, and death. Tolerance builds quickly, and withdrawal is much like detoxification from barbiturates.

Marijuana *Cannabis sativa* is the plant that is used to produce both marijuana and hashish. Marijuana is the unprocessed, dried leaves, flowers, seeds, and stems of the plant. Hashish is stronger, and made from the resin (liquid or semisolid substance) of the plant. Tetrahydrocannabinol (THC) is the strongest psychoactive compound found in cannabis. There are many street names for marijuana: pot, grass, weed, bud, kind

Medical Marijuana

Native Americans have used marijuana medicinally for thousands of years. However, it is illegal in the United States, and the use of marijuana for medical purposes has been extremely controversial. Extensive research has been done on the use of THC to treat people undergoing chemotherapy (a cancer treatment). It has been proven that THC is an effective treatment for the nausea and vomiting associated with this type of cancer treatment. Marijuana also has proven useful for treating glaucoma (an eye disease), wasting syndrome (chronic weight loss and the inability to substantially gain weight once it sets in) associated with AIDS, and other pain syndromes. Marijuana also has been used for asthma relief, spasm relief, anxiety reduction, and relief of alcohol withdrawal symptoms.

At the close of 2012, 18 states—Alaska, Arizona, California, Colorado, Connecticut, Delaware, Hawaii, Maine, Massachusetts, Michigan, Montana, Nevada, New Jersey, New Mexico, Oregon, Rhode Island, Vermont, and Washington, as well as Washington DC had enacted laws legalizing the use of medical marijuana. In 14 of the 18 states patients and/or their caregivers can grow their own marijuana for medicinal use. Home cultivation is not permitted in Connecticut, Delaware, New Jersey, or the District of Columbia, and a special license is required in New Mexico.

Medications based on cannabinoid include manmade compounds, such as dronabinol (Marinol®) and nabilone (Cesamet®), which are FDA approved drugs. A new mixture of THC and cannabidiol called Sativex® is used as a mouth spray and has been approved in Canada and parts of Europe for the relief of cancer-associated pain and pain associated with multiple sclerosis.

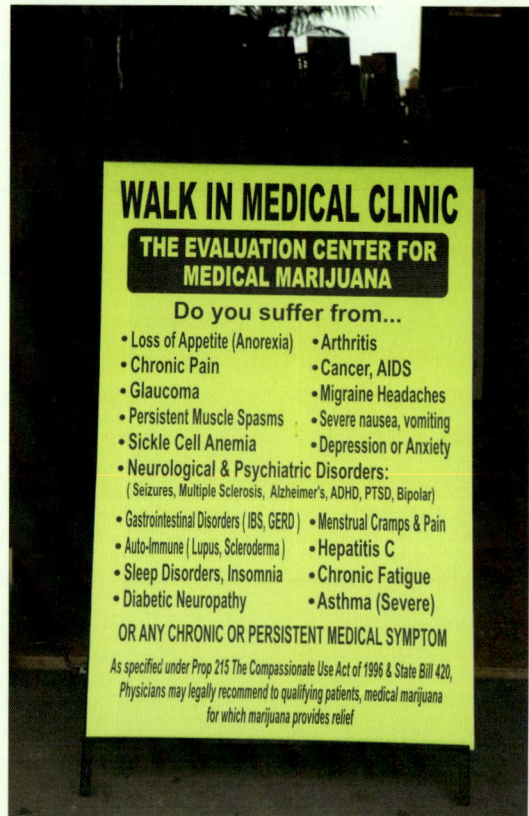

A sign for a local "Walk In Medical Clinic" on the Venice Beach Board Walk in Venice Beach, California, advertises evaluations for the use of medical marijuana. © MIKELEDRAY/ SHUTTERSTOCK.COM.

bud, herb, and reefer are a few. The cigarettes used to roll and smoke the drug are sometimes called doobies, joints, spliffs, fatties, roaches, or blunts. Marijuana can also be smoked in a pipe, or a water pipe, called a bong. In the United States it is the most widely used illicit drug.

The effects of pot often depend on the potency (strength) of the drug. The strength of marijuana has increased tremendously since the 1960s. The common effects of pot smoking are feelings of exhilaration, increased appetite (the "munchies"), relaxation and giddiness (including uncontrollable laughter), increase in heart rate, drowsiness, dry mouth and tongue (referred to as "cotton mouth"), impaired short-term memory, altered perception of time and space, dilated pupils, and paranoia (irrational fear for one's safety). Chronic (frequent) use can cause physical dependence. The long-term adverse effects of marijuana are still unknown, however long-term use commonly leads to addiction and psychological dependence on the drug. Regular users begin to depend on smoking pot to relax and even to sleep. Habitual users often smoke pot immediately upon awakening.

Withdrawal from pot can cause irritability, decreased appetite, sleep disturbances, sweating, nausea, and diarrhea. Hangovers are common the day after smoking pot. They are different from hangovers after drinking alcohol, however. Pot hangovers cause dizziness and inability to concentrate. Marijuana is known to damage the heart and lungs and to suppress the body's immune system. Pot can also make men infertile (unable to father children) and interfere with women's menstrual cycles.

Stimulants

Stimulants are the family of substances that work by increasing the levels of a chemical in the brain associated with pleasure, movement, and attention. They tend to make users feel unusually alert, energetic, and active. Because of their potential for addiction, stimulants are no longer prescribed, as they were in the past, for conditions such as asthma, obesity, and other conditions. Today, they are prescribed to treat just a few specific health conditions, such as attention-deficit / hyperactivity disorder (ADHD), which is a condition marked by difficulty sustaining attention, hyperactivity, and impulsive behavior; narcolepsy, a chronic sleep disorder characterized by overwhelming daytime drowsiness and sudden attacks of sleep; and, less commonly, depression when other treatments have been unsuccessful. The following drugs fall in to the category of stimulants.

Drug use among teenagers has been rising, largely due to increasing use of marijuana. In a 2011 survey, 7% of 8th graders, 18% of 10th graders, and 23% of 12th graders said they had used marijuana in the past month. In the same survey, more than 15% of 12th graders said they had used prescription drugs for non-medical reasons during the past year.

Amphetamines Amphetamines are central nervous system stimulants that give the user a temporary feeling of energy. A popular nickname for amphetamines is "uppers" because they make the user feel up and wide awake. Amphetamines have been used to improve performance—to stay awake, lose weight, or increase concentration—and to get high. When people use them to get high, they generally crush or dissolve them and then snort or inject the mixture.

Therapeutic doses of amphetamines stimulate the central nervous system, increase blood pressure, widen the pupils, quicken the breath, lower appetite, and decrease fatigue. Higher doses can cause agitation, blurred vision, tremors, and heart palpitations. Severe reactions can result in dilated pupils, sweating, cramps, nausea, heart problems, hypertension, panic, aggressive and violent behavior, hallucinations, delirium, high fevers, convulsions, and seizures. People have died from amphetamine abuse because of burst blood vessels, heart attacks, and high fevers. Physical dependence to moderate doses of amphetamines is highly unusual, but psychological dependence from even low doses is common. Chronic users of amphetamines have long-term health consequences. When long-term use of amphetamines is discontinued, withdrawal symptoms may include fatigue, depression, and disturbed sleep patterns.

Methamphetamines Methamphetamine is an amphetamine that can be prescribed by a physician but is rarely prescribed because of its potential for abuse. Most of the methamphetamine sold on the street comes from foreign or U.S. laboratories, although it is also made in small, illegal laboratories, or even in private homes. Methamphetamine is a white, odorless, bitter-tasting crystalline powder that dissolves in water or alcohol and is taken orally, by snorting the powder, by injection, or by smoking. Some street names for it are meth, zip, go-fast, cristy, and chalk. In its crystalline form, the drug is called crystal meth, ice, Tina, or glass. When meth is mixed with water and injected with a needle it is called crank. Sometimes crank is mixed with crack cocaine. The mixture is called "croak."

Methamphetamine abuse changes how the brain functions, and these changes may explain some of the problems users have thinking and controlling their emotions. Taking even small amounts of methamphetamine can produce increased wakefulness, increased physical activity, decreased appetite, increased respiration, and rapid

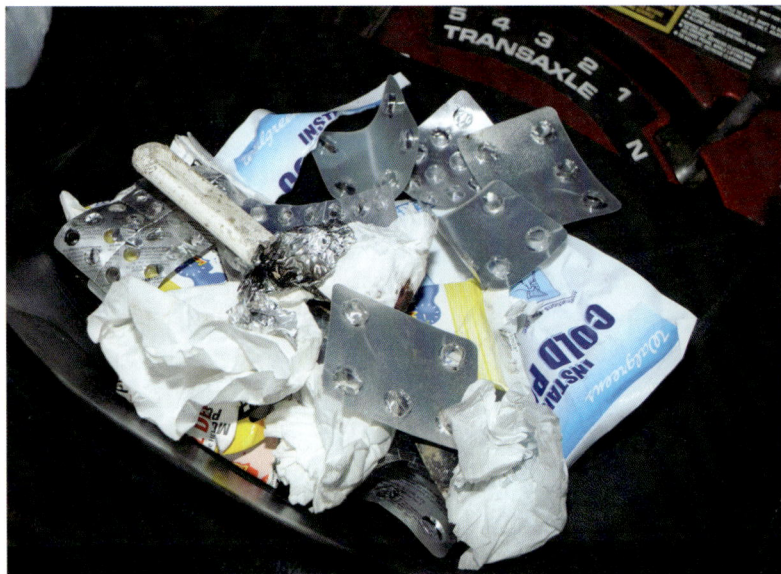

This photo provided by the Franklin County Sheriff's Department shows shake-and-bake meth ingredients found at house that burned from a meth lab explosion in Union, Missouri. Not only is meth bad for those who abuse it, the crude new method of making methamphetamine, by combining raw and unstable ingredients in a 2-liter soda bottle, poses a risk even to those who never get anywhere near the drug. © AP IMAGES/ FRANKLIN COUNTY SHERIFF'S DEPARTMENT.

or irregular heartbeat, as well as increased blood pressure and body temperature.

Over time, methamphetamine abuse can cause many health problems, including extreme weight loss, severe dental problems, anxiety, confusion, sleeplessness, mood disturbances, and violent behavior. Chronic methamphetamine abusers also may become paranoid (extreme, irrational fear or mistrust of others), have hallucinations, or experience delusions, such as the feeling that they can fly or that insects are crawling under their skin.

Crystal meth is even more dangerous than the typical, older forms of amphetamines because it gets into the system faster, lasts longer, and can have even more deadly effects. In addition to tremors and convulsions, increased blood pressure, irregular heart rate, and intense anxiety, users also may have mood swings and violent thoughts and behavior.

Cocaine Cocaine is another central nervous system stimulant. It comes from the coca plant, found in South America. (From 1891 to 1903,

Clubs and Drugs

A very pure form of methamphetamine may be smoked in a pipe. In this form, the drug looks like little chips of ice. For that reason, it has been called ice, glass, or crystal meth. Ravers, young people that go to all-night dance parties, often use it. Raves are parties where electronic music is played and drugs such as meth, acid (LSD, or lysergic acid diethylamide), and ecstasy (MDMA, or methylenedioxymethlamphetamine) are common and easily available. Party goers who want to stay awake and dance until the sunrise (and often beyond) often use meth.

the soft drink Coca-Cola contained extracts of the coca leaf.) Some street names for cocaine are blow, C, coke, and snow. It is usually snorted but also may be injected or smoked. At one time, cocaine was very expensive, and only the very wealthy could buy it. Crack is a form of cocaine that is smoked; it is much more potent (strong), cheaper, and sold in rocks. Crack is highly addictive; some experts say even one use has the potential to make someone addicted.

Cocaine causes an initial euphoric high that can last from 15 to 30 minutes. People on cocaine tend to talk rapidly and feel like they are invincible. Socially awkward people on cocaine jump out of their shells and act tremendously self-confident, often arrogant. A cocaine user may feel sexually stimulated at first, but as the drug wears off this usually doesn't last.

The high from cocaine is short-lived, and "crashing" quickly sets in. A person crashing from a cocaine high is usually depressed, paranoid, irritable, and extremely tired. Because the high is so brief, cocaine users tend to buy a large amount of the drug and go through it quickly. Cocaine has the reputation of being a social drug, and people tend to do it with groups in bars and clubs. For serious users, cocaine binges can last for days. On a binge, a user will snort cocaine every half-hour for days on end. They will live without sleep or food until they crash from exhaustion.

Cocaine is highly addicting, although it is not physically addictive in the way that narcotics, such as heroin, can be. That is, physical tolerance to cocaine does not develop. Rather, users need to take it again and again to avoid crashing. Even one-time use of cocaine can result in death.

PCP PCP (phencyclidine) is a man-made drug that alters people's perceptions of sight and sound and makes users feel distanced and detached. Also known as angel dust, it usually looks like white or colored chunks, powder, or crystals. It is often smoked but also may be snorted or eaten. Low doses produce muscle stiffness and poor coordination, slurred speech, drowsiness, confusion, numbness of the arms and legs, profuse sweating, nausea, vomiting, flushing, and increased heart rate. Strange and violent behavior can result from higher doses. In some cases effects from PCP have lasted up to 10 weeks. Heavy users can experience deep anxiety, depression, and psychotic symptoms.

Hallucinogens

Hallucinogens or psychedelics were the most popular class of drugs in the 1960s. Timothy Leary (1920–1996), a doctor from Harvard University, coined the phrase, "Tune in, turn on, drop out," encouraging young people everywhere to experiment with psychedelics. Hallucinogens affect people by distorting reality, and, at higher doses, often cause hallucinations (the illusion of seeing or hearing something that isn't really present). (Other drugs, even alcohol and marijuana, can cause hallucinations, too.)

Synthetic hallucinogens are LSD (lysergic acid diethylamide), mescaline (peyote), and DOM and STP (2,5-dimethoxy-4-methylamphetamine), an amphetamine derivative. LSD is also called acid. Synthetic hallucinogens are manufactured in underground laboratories that exist only to serve the illegal drug market. Natural hallucinogens include buttons from the peyote cactus (the active ingredient, mescaline, can also be synthetically produced), morning glory seeds, and psilocybin mushrooms (these are often called "shrooms" or "magic mushrooms"; they are not the kind of mushrooms found in supermarkets).

The slang term for taking hallucinogens is "tripping." The experience an individual can have on psychedelics varies widely. The emotional and mental state of the user at the time of "dropping" or taking the drug sets the tone for the trip. If the individual has any feelings of doubt or fear, the drug often exaggerates these emotions. This can cause a nightmarish experience, called a "bad trip." Trips can last anywhere from four to 24 hours depending on dosage and circumstances.

LSD. LSD can be taken in different forms. Because it is highly potent, only small amounts are necessary. It is sometimes produced in pill form. More commonly, sheets of LSD called blotter paper are produced. The user puts a tiny piece of the sheet in his or her mouth. These pieces are called dots, tabs, or doses. Sometimes acid is taken in liquid form. The effects of LSD are usually felt within an hour. Physical effects include increased blood pressure, dilated pupils, rapid heartbeat, muscular weakness, trembling, nausea, chills, and hyperventilation. (Sometimes LSD is mixed with amphetamines, and the effects match the speedy physical effects of that class of drugs.) Another possible effect of taking LSD is the flashback. Up to a year after the acid trip, users may have hallucinations caused by LSD left in their systems.

Mescaline. Mescaline is made from the peyote cactus. The heads or "buttons" of the cactus are dried and put into capsules. It is usually taken orally but also may be smoked or injected. It is less potent than LSD. Physical effects include dilated pupils, high body temperature, nausea and vomiting, and muscular relaxation. Mental effects include euphoria, heightened sensory perception, hallucinations, and difficulty in thinking. Higher doses can cause headaches, dry skin, hypotension (lowering of the blood pressure), cardiac depression, and slowing of respiration.

Designer Drugs Designer drugs, called such because they are "designed" in a laboratory, were created in the 1970s by underground chemists attempting to subvert the drug laws of the day. The designer drugs were only a molecule or two different than some of the synthetic drugs then listed as illegal according to the Controlled Substance Act.

Ecstasy (MDMA) MDMA, better known as Ecstasy, is a very popular designer drug. Some street names for Ecstasy are X, E, XTC, Rave, or Adam. It is related to amphetamines and mescaline. It is also called the "love drug" or the "hug drug" because it enhances empathy and relatedness. It also causes a positive mood change, a drop in defense mechanisms, and elevated mood. Some of the negative effects of Ecstasy are the potential for overdosing, extreme fatigue, dilated pupils, dry mouth and throat, tension in the lower jaw, grinding of the teeth, and overstimulation. It can also cause extreme paranoia and panic that call for emergency care.

Ketamine Ketaminehydrochloride is another potentially deadly designer drug. It is a drug widely used as an animal tranquilizer by veterinarians during surgery. Also known as Special K or vitamin K, it is made by drying ketamine (often in a stove) until it turns from a liquid to a white, crystalline powder. It is a very powerful hallucinogen. It is usually snorted, but it is sometimes sprinkled on tobacco or marijuana cigarettes and smoked. Ketamine is frequently used in combination with other drugs, such as Ecstasy, heroin, and cocaine.

People high on ketamine may have profound hallucinations that include visual distortions and a lost sense of time, sense, and identity. Users report having profoundly terrifying experiences while high. Some report experiencing total temporary paralysis (loss of the ability to move or feel sensation). The high lasts anywhere from a half hour to two hours. Because users generally become unable to speak or even see what is happening around them, it is not a social drug. Like other designer drugs, ketamine is often cut with other drugs and poisonous agents.

Bath Salts In 2010, awareness grew of several new synthetic stimulants packaged and marketed as "bath salts" (or sometimes "plant food"). The name bath salts comes from the white, crystalline form of the drug, which resembles legally sold salts used in bathing products, however the drugs are unrelated to such salts. Bath salts are found in head shops (stores where drug paraphernalia is sold), gas stations, and on the Internet under names such as "Zoom," "Ivory Wave," "Purple Wave," "Cloud Nine," "Vanilla Sky," or "Bliss," and are thus easy to access and inexpensive, leading to use by adolescents and teens. The drug is usually swallowed or smoked (though it can also be snorted or injected) to obtain a high similar to that of cocaine or amphetamines. Side effects can include headaches, panic attacks, agitation, paranoia, hallucinations, violent behavior, and even death.

The packages state that the products are not for human consumption in an effort to avoid being labeled as illegal drugs, and the makers of the products constantly tinker with the ingredients used to keep one step ahead of the authorities. However, after increasing reports of poisonings related to bath salts in 2011, the DEA banned three of the synthetic stimulants—Mephedrone, 3,4 methylenedioxypyrovalerone (MDPV), and Methylone—used to make such products. In 2012, Congress passed and President Obama signed the Synthetic Drug Abuse Prevention Act to ban dozens of different chemicals used to make the drugs. The act does not name specific recipes, so that all synthetic drugs like bath salts are covered.

Spice Another recent designer drug is a synthetic version of marijuana commonly called spice, K2, incense, or potpourri, which, like bath salts, was sold legally on the Internet and in places like malls, convenience stores, and gas stations. The chemicals in such products are usually manufactured in China and then sprayed on incense that can be burned or leaves that can be smoked or made into a tea, leading to

"Smiles" Is a Deadly Hallucinogen

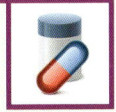

In 2012 several teenagers died after using an illegal man-made drug called 2C-I that also is known as "Smiles." 2C-I is one of a group of compounds that cause users to hallucinate. 2C-I is also similar to a class of drugs that are related to amphetamines. As a result, in addition to relaxation and hallucinations, users may have increased heart rates and irregular heart rhythms. They also may suffer from nausea and vomiting and overwhelming fear and panic. Usually sold in powder form, users often mix the powder with chocolate or candy before consuming it. 2C-I can also be taken as a tablet.

a psychoactive high. Side effects can include vomiting, hallucinations, agitation, increased sweating, inability to talk, memory loss, high blood pressure, psychosis, violent behaviors, and death. As with bath salts, the manufacturers tried to stay one step ahead of the authorities by changing ingredients to keep the drugs legal, which means that the high and the side effects may be different each time someone uses a different formulation of the drug. However, the Synthetic Drug Abuse Prevention Act signed into law in 2012 now covers these products as well as bath salts.

Inhalants

Inhalants are chemical vapors that people sniff to get high. The sniffing of glue, solvents, aerosols, cleaning agents, gas from dessert topping sprays, and other gases is another means people use to achieve a high. Because common, everyday products found in most homes and grocery stores can be used as inhalants, sniffing, also called huffing, is popular with teens and others who don't have money or access to buy illegal drugs. People who use inhalants are sometimes referred to as "huffers."

Because the inhalants are legal, everyday products, many teens do not view sniffing as being as harmful as doing "hard" drugs. This is a dangerous and untrue belief. Symptoms of inhalant use are slurred speech, mental disorientation, headaches, dizziness and weakness, muscle spasms, euphoria, and nystagmus (eye movement from side to side). Some of the more serious adverse effects are nausea and vomiting, confusion, panic, tension, aggressive behavior, and permanent brain damage. At higher doses, use of inhalants can cause respiratory depression, heart failure, and loss of consciousness, resulting in coma and death.

Alcohol and Alcoholism

Alcohol is classified as a central nervous system depressant like barbiturates and tranquilizers. Although it is legal for persons of over age 21 in the United States to use, it is still very much a drug. It is, however, a socially acceptable drug, unlike some of the drugs already discussed. After tobacco, alcohol is the most widely used psychoactive drug in the world.

Drinking alcohol, whether beer, wine, or liquor, causes a vast array of effects. Even small amounts of alcohol impair drinkers so much that they cannot perform simple motor tasks. Every tissue in the human body is affected by alcohol consumption. Individual effects of drinking vary. Body weight and size, sex, metabolism, the amount of alcohol consumed

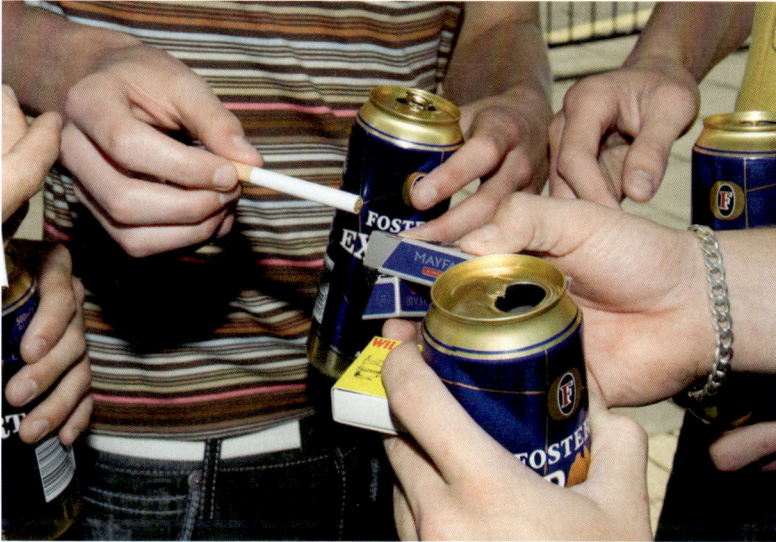

at the time, and the type and amount of food in the stomach determine the blood alcohol level. Mild intoxication can cause feelings of warmth, flushed skin, impaired judgment, and decreased inhibitions. Deeper intoxication can cause a slowing of reflexes and more obvious lessening of judgment and inhibitions. Slurred speech, double vision, and memory and comprehension loss can follow.

Drinkers may experience vomiting, incontinence (losing bladder or bowel control), and the inability to stand on their own. Many people pass out when they've had too much to drink. Blackouts are not uncommon. In a blackout, drinkers will not remember large segments of their experiences. Coma and death are possible results of excessive drinking. Drinking even a small amount of alcohol can result in a hangover. Hangovers can cause headaches, fatigue, nausea, shakiness, and extreme thirst. (For those who insist on drinking, consuming plenty of water before, during, and after will prevent the dehydration that is a consequence of alcohol consumption.)

Alcohol abuse is when drinking causes problems in people's lives. Short-term abuse can cause the physical reactions described above, along with the possibility of serious hazards incurred by loss of faculties. Drunk driving is the most serious and immediate consequence. Drunk people may make bad decisions that can cost them their lives and the lives of those they love. The decision to get behind the wheel after drinking can result in drivers having to spend the rest of their lives in prison. Death is

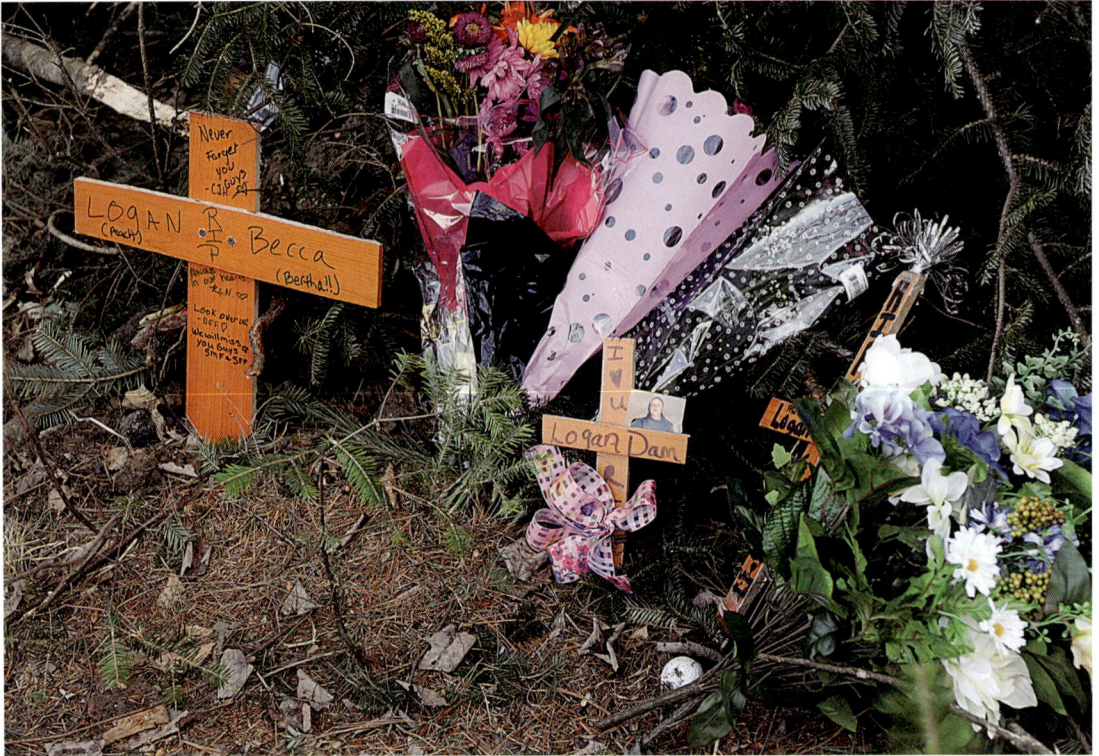

Flowers placed by friends and family members of two teens are seen at the site of the auto accident that killed them both. The driver was drinking and texting while driving. Alcohol impairs reflexes and slows response times, and when coupled with trying to text, can be deadly for the driver and others. © AP IMAGES/SUN JOURNAL/AMBER WATERMAN.

the most serious result of driving drunk. People who have been drinking, even those who do not think they are drunk, should never drive, no matter the circumstances.

Alcohol can be addictive. The physical and psychological need for alcohol can turn into a chronic disease known as alcoholism. People suffering from alcoholism cannot keep from drinking and cannot stop drinking even though they know that they are harming their health and their lives. Alcoholism runs in families, and researchers believe that certain genes may increase the risk of alcoholism, but it is not yet known exactly which genes increase susceptibility to alcoholism.

Long-term effects of alcohol abuse and alcoholism include liver diseases, such as cirrhosis, and cancer. These are usually fatal. Alcoholics have higher rates of peptic ulcers, pneumonia, cancer of the upper digestive and respiratory tracts, heart and artery disease, tuberculosis, and suicide than the rest of the population. Fetal alcohol syndrome (FAS) is a condition that drinking mothers pass on to their infants. Pregnant women should not drink alcohol at all. FAS is the leading cause of birth defects.

Withdrawal from Alcohol Six to 12 hours after the last drink, an alcoholic can begin to feel the effects of withdrawal from alcohol. The stage one symptoms are psychomotor agitation, anxiety, insomnia, appetite suppression, stomach problems, elevated heart rate and blood pressure, sweating and tremors. Within 24 hours, stage two withdrawal symptoms begin. They include the symptoms of stage one, plus hallucinations and seizures.

Nicotine

Nicotine is an addictive drug that is legal in the United States for persons over the age of 18. It is found in tobacco products, most notably cigarettes. Although the law prohibits selling cigarettes to minors, smoking is common among teens. Many people do not think of cigarettes

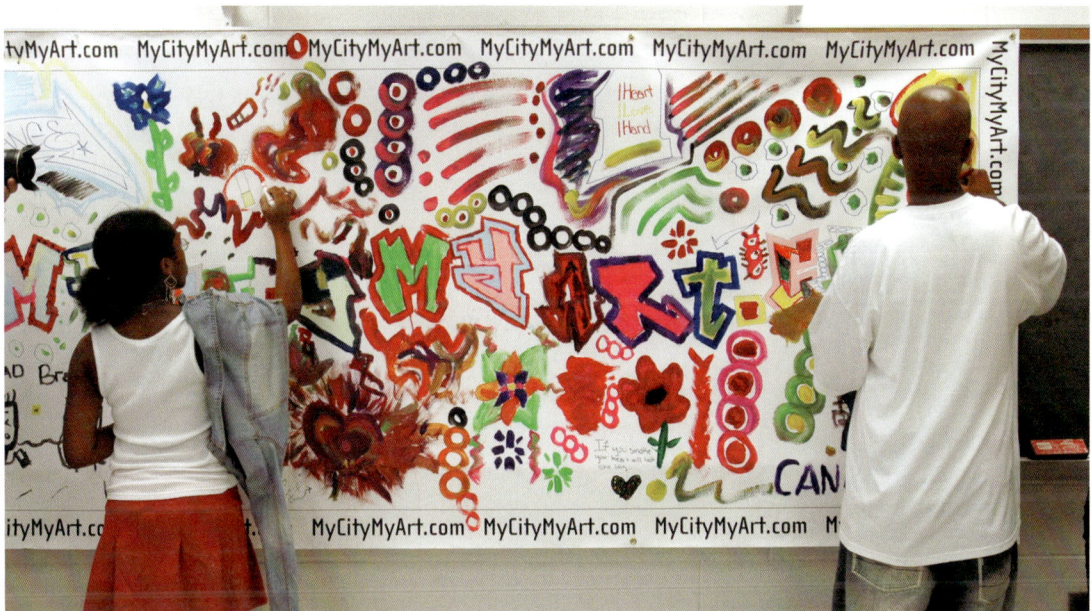

Children from the Philadelphia charity CORA Services join graffiti artist Pose2 in creating an oversized stop-smoking themed mural. This is part of Nicorette nicotine gums' effort to help raise awareness in the African American community about how adults can stop smoking and why children should never start. © AP IMAGES/PRNEWSFOTO/GLAXOSMITHKLINE.

as drugs but smoking is the most lethal of all the addictive behaviors. Smoking kills more people each year than AIDS, fires, illegal drugs, and suicides combined. It is best to avoid smoking altogether because it is among the most difficult addictions to shake.

Smoking causes coughing, shortness of breath, fatigue, yellow teeth, bad breath, heart disease, lung cancer, throat and mouth cancer, dry skin, dry hair, emphysema (a chronic lung disease), asthma, and a variety of other problems. At one time, the dangers of nicotine and smoking were not as well known as they are today, and smoking was a symbol of "being cool." That era is long gone. And the proven negative effects of smoking are well documented. Pregnant and breast-feeding women face special risks and dangers when it comes to smoking. For example, a fetus exposed to the effects of smoking runs the risk of having a low birth weight.

Caffeine

Caffeine is a stimulant found in coffee, some teas, chocolate, some over-the-counter drugs, energy drinks, and cola drinks. Due to the popularity of these products, especially coffee and cola drinks, caffeine is the most popular drug in the world. It is sometimes used medically, but mostly caffeine is used non-medically for its stimulating effect on mood and behavior. When someone wakes up in the morning and can't get started without a cup of coffee, this is a classic sign of caffeine addiction. People who regularly consume five or more cups of coffee per day develop a tolerance to caffeine. Withdrawal from caffeine or even a reduction in the amount consumed may cause headache, irritability, and drowsiness.

About one-quarter of U.S. high school students smoke cigarettes, and 8% use smokeless tobacco. About 30% of teens who smoke will continue to smoke as adults and will die early from a smoking-related disease. People who start smoking as teenagers have the hardest time quitting.

Treatment for Addiction

Whether a person is suffering from alcoholism, nicotine addiction, or drug addiction, treatment is necessary for successful recovery. Going "cold turkey," the idea of abruptly quitting using a substance without any treatment, only works for a very small minority. Many people believe in the saying "once an addict, always an addict." That is, recovery from addiction is thought to be a lifelong process and not one that stops once an addict initially stops using. Many former addicts who have been substance-free for years still consider themselves in recovery. There are many options available for people seeking help to recover from addictions.

Alcoholics Anonymous (AA) Alcoholics Anonymous (AA) is the most famous treatment organization in the world. AA meetings take place just about everywhere in the United States each day and in other countries as well. AA is based on a 12-step recovery plan. These are the steps successful members of AA completed:

1. We admitted we were powerless over alcohol—that our lives had become unmanageable.

2. Came to believe that a Power greater than ourselves could restore us to sanity.

3. Made a decision to turn our will and our lives over to the care of God, as we understood Him.

4. Made a searching and fearless moral inventory of ourselves.

5. Admitted to God, to ourselves and to another human being the exact nature of our wrongs.

6. Were entirely ready to have God remove all these defects of character.

7. Humbly asked Him to remove our shortcomings.

8. Made a list of all persons we had harmed, and became willing to make amends to them all.

9. Made direct amends to such people wherever possible, except when to do so would injure them or others.

10. Continued to take personal inventory, and when we were wrong, promptly admitted it.

11. Sought through prayer and meditation to improve our conscious contact with God, as we understood Him, praying only for knowledge of His will for us and the power to carry that out.

12. Having had a spiritual awakening as the result of these steps, we tried to carry this message to alcoholics and to practice these principles in all our affairs.

Sugar Addiction

The average American consumes about 22 teaspoons of sugar a day, which is about 100 pounds of sugar each year. Sugar addiction is common among children and adults and is no different, in terms of physical response, than addiction to other substances. Refined white sugar is an ingredient in almost all processed foods found at the supermarket: breakfast cereals, sodas, breads, canned soups, cakes, cookies, ice cream, and many other food products. It is in just about everything but raw fruits and vegetables (which contain natural, not refined, sugar).

Sugar consumption has a powerful effect on the human body. It causes insulin (a hormone that regulates the amount of sugar in the blood) in the body to rise, and energy temporarily shoots up. That is why people sometimes reach for candy bars when they need a quick lift. But the problem with the rise in energy is the consequent crash. Once the sugar leaves the system, the sugar-eater gets fatigued and craves more. This causes a cycle of dependence that is hard to break. Because refined white sugar is a food (and because it's hard to avoid unless one really makes an effort) most people do not connect health and emotional problems to sugar addiction (for instance, some hyperactive children return to normal behavior when taken off sugar). In the long run, too much processed sugar can cause cavities, increase risk for diabetes, and contribute to a host of other illnesses.

Take the Quiz

On its web site (http://www.alcoholics-anonymous.org) Alcoholics Anonymous has a questionnaire for teens. If teens take the quiz and answer even one question with a "yes," they are directed to explore whether they might have a serious problem with alcohol.

A Simple 12-Question Quiz Designed To Help You Decide

1. Do you drink because you have problems? To relax?

2. Do you drink when you get mad at other people, your friends or parents?

3. Do you prefer to drink alone, rather than with others?

4. Are your grades starting to slip? Are you goofing off on your job?

5. Did you ever try to stop drinking or drink less—and fail?

6. Have you begun to drink in the morning, before school or work?

7. Do you gulp your drinks?

8. Do you ever have loss of memory due to your drinking?

9. Do you lie about your drinking?

10. Do you ever get into trouble when you're drinking?

11. Do you get drunk when you drink, even when you don't mean to?

12. Do you think it's cool to be able to hold your liquor?

These steps have been modified and used by many other recovery programs for all different types of addictions. AA is a plan for self-reflection and taking responsibility. Some people are uncomfortable with the word God, and the reference to God as a Him. Those individuals can substitute other words for any spiritual language, and the steps can still work for them.

Abstinence from all alcohol is a requirement for those in AA. New members are given a sponsor, a recovering alcoholic (called such because many former alcoholics feel they are always in recovery) who can lead them through the process. The sponsor stands by to assist the new members. If they feel they might relapse (that is, return to drinking), they are told to call their sponsor right away for guidance.

Methadone Maintenance Methadone maintenance is a popular treatment for heroin addicts. Methadone is a substitute drug for heroin. It is prescribed and distributed in a controlled environment. It helps to relieve the severe symptoms of withdrawal from heroin, without enforcing abstinence. The goal of methadone maintenance is to wean a heroin addict from heroin and then, ultimately, from methadone, which does not have as severe withdrawal symptoms as does heroin. Widespread HIV infection among heroin addicts (from sharing dirty needles) increased the acceptance of methadone maintenance as a treatment for addiction in the United States. (European countries have used this treatment for years without problems.)

Intervention Intervention is a popular mode of treatment for addiction and other behavioral problems. Intervention is an organized visit upon the afflicted individual by friends and loved ones. Often a counselor is present, and counselors almost always help to plan the meeting.

The intervention is designed to confront the person suffering from addiction in a nonjudgmental fashion. Group members tell the individual that they are aware of the addiction and that they care for the person and want him or her to seek help and get better. Often an intervention helps addicts realize that their addiction is not a secret and that they are affecting their friends' and loved ones' lives. An intervention also may backfire, causing the subject of the intervention to become immediately defensive and storm out of the meeting. That is why taking this approach needs to be considered very carefully and should involve a trained substance abuse counselor.

Other Treatment Considerations Anyone suffering from addiction and attempting to recover will experience a certain degree of pain and discomfort. The person must believe that kicking the habit is worth it and be willing to ride out the discomfort to reach sobriety. While this is much easier said than done, there are some tools that recovering addicts can use to ease the road to recovery.

It makes sense for all people to eat healthful diets and get enough sleep, but for people that have been abusing their bodies with a substance, healthy eating is even more important. Regular exercise is also vital for the recovering person.

Acupuncture. Acupuncture is used to help ward off cravings. Acupuncture is an ancient Chinese method of placing very thin needles in strategic points on the body. The points correspond to energy meridians, and they restore balance to the body. Ear point acupuncture is often offered in methadone clinics for heroin addicts.

Meditation. Meditation is focusing intently on one sound, idea, image, or goal. For a person recovering from addiction, meditation may be extremely difficult but it can be extremely valuable. When someone stops to look at waves crashing on the beach or a candle flame or even a tree in the park, often that person will enter into a trance-like state. This is a form of meditation. Artists of all types often become so

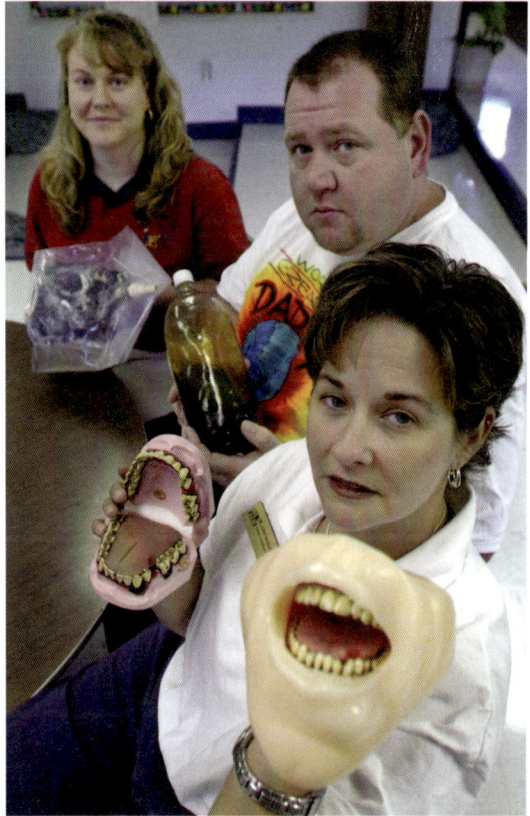

High school staff hold visual aids, a diseased human lung, a bottle full of the tar accumulated in the lungs by a pack-a-day smoker in just one year, and models of the mouth of a smokeless tobacco user and the mouth of smoker. The three use the visual aids while conducting an eight week smoking awareness program followed by an eight week smoking cessation program for 14 students at the school. © AP IMAGES/ GARY EMORD-NETZLEY.

How to Meditate

The first thing one needs to do is find a safe, quiet space where one will not be disturbed. (Meditation in bed is not recommended.) Sometimes people use a meditation cushion to sit on (this can simply be a pillow or couch cushion). Comfort is essential for meditation. Sitting in a chair, or against the wall if this is more comfortable, is fine, too. Having the feet fall asleep can get in the way of the practice.

Meditation begins by breathing. Breathing should be natural, and one should try to be aware of each breath taken. Then the mantra should be repeated, over and over, slowly, in the mind. Obsessive thoughts may creep into the mind during meditation. Meditation teachers suggest that those starting a practice should try to let their thoughts go and use the metaphor of the movie screen. Some people like to pretend that their mind is a movie screen and that the thoughts passing are not their own. This is a good way to detach from painful thoughts. When people try to control their thoughts, or punish themselves for their thoughts, they have trouble with meditation. Gentle return to the mantra is suggested when thoughts stray. It is important not to get frustrated because thoughts will naturally stray. Twenty minutes per session is usually recommended, but five minutes is good for a starting practice. Healing may not be immediate with meditation, but recovering people who have learned to meditate report tremendous benefits from their practice.

involved in the act of making art that it becomes a meditation.

Concentration is one of the most difficult tasks for recovering addicts. Thoughts and obsessions run like wildfire through the mind. Meditating is like going on vacation in the mind even while the body is stuck in one spot. Meditation also helps with insomnia (sleeplessness), a problem for many recovering people. Meditation before bed (but not in bed) helps to create deep and peaceful sleep.

Mantras. A mantra is simply a sound, word, or phrase that is repeated over and over during meditation. Many people think the best mantras are the ones that have no distinct meaning, the ones that are simply sounds. (For instance, the sound "ohm" is a popular choice.) This is so that the meditator will not begin thinking about meditation. The goal of meditation is to go to a place of focus where passing, disturbed thoughts do not interfere with relaxation.

The most important factors in healing from addiction are honesty and love of self. Without those fundamental foundations, no treatment plan can work. Once the person with an addiction admits to being sick and needing help, he or she is ready to begin the long road to feeling whole again. The addiction has likely become a great comfort to the addict, something he believes he can't do without. Giving up that idea and letting go of the substance itself is not easy, but it can be done. Just as getting hooked changes people's lives, they can change again, for the better, by recovering from their addictions.

Compulsive Behaviors

Compulsions are habitual behaviors or mental acts a person is driven to perform in order to reduce stress and anxiety. Psychological vulnerability,

Healthy Living, 2nd Edition

cultural and social factors, as well as contact with others engaging in compulsive behaviors all influence the development of compulsive behaviors. It is important to note that any of the following activities or behaviors in moderation is fine. However, when a normal activity becomes one in which the person is trapped in a pattern of repetitive behaviors he or she cannot control, it is considered a compulsion.

Gambling Gambling can be a dangerous compulsion. Compulsive gamblers often spend all their money, exhaust their savings, and even resort to stealing money to support their habits. People can become addicted to betting on sports events, playing poker, or playing slot machines in bars and casinos. Something about the possibility of winning, perhaps the risk and the consequent adrenaline rush, spur on compulsive gamblers. Virtual casinos and online gambling sites are immediately available to those who cannot travel to popular gambling destinations like Las Vegas, Nevada, or Atlantic City, New Jersey. Easy online access to gambling has increased the numbers of teens that gamble. Unlike actual casinos, the Web sites do not require proof of age or an ID. As a result, the underage gamblers can gain instant access to virtual casinos.

The Center for Online Addiction (www.netaddiction.com) exists to serve people with all forms of Internet addiction, including addiction to online gambling. Addiction to online auction houses, such as ebay, is another form of compulsive gambling.

Internet Addiction Internet addiction is a broad term that describes many kinds of compulsive behaviors. Many potentially addictive activities in real life are replicated on the Internet. The reason Internet addictions are a bit more dangerous is that people often feel secluded sitting in front of their computer screens. There is a sense that they won't get caught in the act.

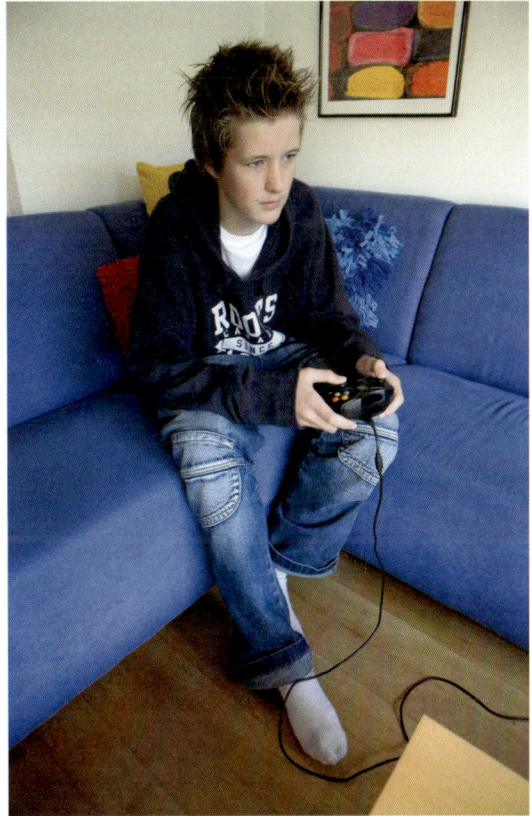

Playing video games and using the Internet can be fun distractions, but computer addiction can occur. If a person starts to play video games compulsively or becomes addicted to various activities on the Internet, counseling may be suggested to help the person reintegrate with society. © PICTURE PARTNERS/ALAMY.

According the Center for Online Addiction, there are different types of Internet addiction:

- Cyber-sexual addiction is an addiction to adult chat rooms or cyber-porn.
- Cyber-relationship addiction is addiction to meeting people on the Internet, usually in chat rooms or through newsgroups. People who grow addicted to meeting people in the virtual world often stop seeing and speaking to their friends from real life.
- Net compulsions are the gambling related activities described above.
- Information overload is compulsive Web surfing and researching. Sometimes information overload can keep people up all night surfing, which may leave them to tired for their normal daily activities.
- General computer addiction describes those who compulsively play video games or program their computers.

People who hide out in a cyber universe are often troubled and have difficulty socializing with real people. Counseling may help Internet addicts come out from behind their computers and rejoin the real world.

Exercise Addiction Exercise addiction is compulsive exercise that harms rather than improves people's health. People addicted to exercise think about exercise constantly and plan their every moment around the next time they can run, bike, take a class at the gym, or lift weights. They talk constantly about fitness. They begin to associate only with those people who will indulge their addiction: people who also exercise all the time. If someone gets really angry or depressed by missing a workout, or if he or she constantly exercises and stops taking part in other social activities, that individual might be an exercise addict.

Exercise addiction can lead to exhaustion and even death. Women may stop getting their periods, and men who are obsessed with muscles sometimes succumb to taking dangerous steroids to bulk up. For most people, a new exercise regimen, often under the supervision of a doctor or a trainer, is truly beneficial for their health. But in some cases, the healthful benefits of exercise are lost and replaced with the desperate need to exercise all the time.

Often exercise addiction is related to body image disorders, like anorexia nervosa, bulimia nervosa, and body dysmorphic disorder. In all three of these illnesses, people see themselves not as they are, but as a distorted, fat people who do not measure up to society's standards of thinness or fitness. (In the case of body dysmorphic disorder, fat is not always the culprit but rather a constant unhappiness with parts of, or the shape of, one's body.) Women and girls tend to suffer from this kind of disease most often, but increasing numbers of boys and men are affected too.

Exercise addiction can develop for other reasons as well. For instance, athletes can become addicted to training in their quest to improve their performance. Abuse of steroids can occur along with exercise addiction. Steroids are a class of drugs that increase the male hormone testosterone in the body. This increases muscle mass when accompanied by weight training. In the weight lifting world, there is a focus on looking "buff" or very muscular. Many men (and women, too) who weight train sometimes become so focused on the goal of attaining huge muscles that they turn to steroids as a means of bulking up.

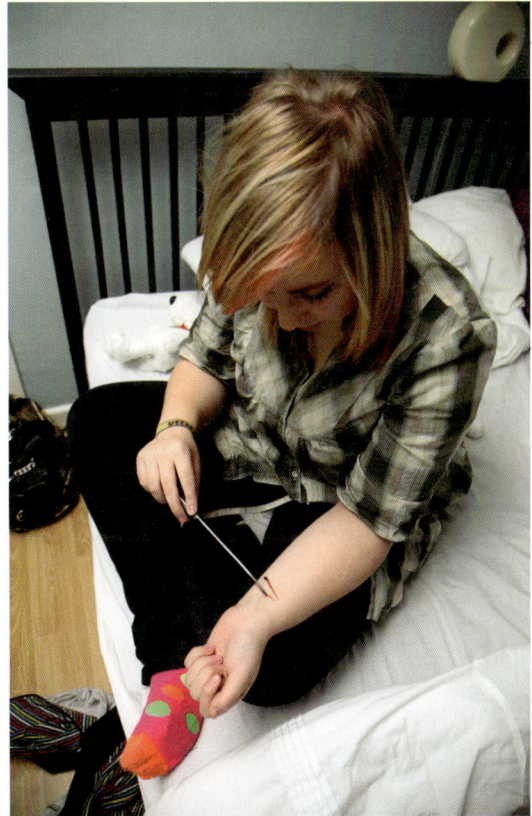

Self harm, such as cutting, burning, hitting oneself, head banging, or hair pulling may be signs of a depression, personality disorder, or other disorder. Some people who self harm may also be suicidal.
© LEILA CUTLER/ALAMY.

Self-Injury Self-injury or self-harm, often expressed by cutting or burning oneself, is considered an impulse-control behavior problem, but also may be symptom of another mental health disorder such as depression, a personality disorder, or it may occur along with an eating disorder. It is a dangerous, unhealthy way to deal with emotional problems such as pain, anger, and frustration. Self-injury may give people a brief moment of relief, but the painful emotions that caused it quickly return.

Self-injury is common among teenage girls, but anyone can develop this dangerous behavior. Those who self harm sometimes carve on their body with razor blades, stick themselves with pins, and squeeze and pinch their faces.

It is very important that people who self-injure receive therapy to uncover the reasons they are hurting themselves. Therapy aims to help people manage the issues that trigger the behavior. Recovering from self-injury may take a long time because it may have become a major part of a person's life and because it may be a symptom of another mental disorder.

Manias A mania is an excessive or unreasonable enthusiasm for an activity, especially a destructive activity such as stealing or starting fires. Low levels of serotonin, a naturally occurring chemical in the brain, are common in people prone to impulsive behaviors.

Kleptomania is the compulsion to steal. Kleptomaniacs lead dangerous lives, stealing things every chance they get. It's not enough for them to simply shoplift from stores. Kleptomaniacs steal from their friends, teachers, and loved ones. Like other behaviors involving risk, the risk of getting caught seems to satisfy some need in people who compulsively steal.

Pyromaniacs are people that feel compelled to start fires. This compulsion not only may kill the person who sets the fire, but also anyone caught in the way. Experts believe that some firesetters may be seeking attention while others are thrill-seekers. Teens who set fires often have committed other crimes such as vandalism or sexual offenses. Pyromaniacs are often angry people, but the anger is often suppressed. Setting fires is a way for them to express their anger. Usually pyromaniacs don't get help until it is too late. A serious fire is often the event that forces them into therapy.

Compulsive Shopping Compulsive shopping is an addiction that causes people to run up their credit card bills and get so buried in debt that they sometimes have to declare bankruptcy (legally declare themselves unable to pay their bills due to lack of money). Many people, at one time or another, purchase an item that they do not really need or want. Compulsive shoppers, however, go on frequent shopping sprees and buy many things that they just don't need at all. Somehow, standing in front of the item before they buy it, they believe that their lives will be better if they own the item. As a result, they end up with closets full of unnecessary items.

Compulsive shoppers are searching for love in the form of material objects. They experience tension or anxiety before they make a purchase, and a sense of relief following the purchase. Often they continue shopping until a loved one stops them or they lose everything to debt. Compulsive shopping tends to run in families, and many people with this disorder also suffer from depression, anxiety, substance abuse disorders, and eating disorders.

Sex Addiction Sex addiction is the compulsion to repeatedly seek out people and have sexual relations with them. Sex addicts put themselves in dangerous situations regularly just to fulfill their need to have sex. People who are sex addicts sometimes meet strangers in bars, or almost anywhere, and go some place with that stranger to engage in casual sexual activity. Of course, when a stranger is involved there is a great deal of danger from potential personal harm. People who engage in such behaviors are not just being promiscuous; rather, they are psychologically driven by their sex addiction.

Sex addiction is treatable. Once addicts confront and accept their behavior, they can begin to look at the reasons why they are compelled to have sex all the time. Often sex addicts experienced sexual abuse (when a person is forced to engage in sexual activities against his or her will) as children. Their sex addiction is a way of having control over their bodies and the act of seduction they compulsively perform is a way of controlling a partner. Sex addiction is never connected to healthy love and desire.

Most sex addicts deny their addiction, and successful treatment of addiction requires that people admit that they have a problem. Often, a crisis—such as the loss of a job, the end of a marriage, or illness—must occur before sex addicts seek treatment. Treatment focuses on controlling the addictive behavior and helping the person develop a healthy sexuality. Support groups and 12 step recovery programs for people with sexual addictions, such as Sex Addicts Anonymous, help many people to recover.

Eating Disorders

Eating disorders are dangerous psychological (relating to the mind) illnesses that affect millions of people, especially young women and girls. Many experts describe eating disorders as addictions. The most widely known eating disorders are anorexia nervosa, bulimia nervosa, and binge eating disorder, in which people eat abnormally large quantities of food in short periods of time.

Eating Disorders Named

English physician Richard Morton first documented cases of self-starvation in the 17th century. French neurologist Charles Lasegue and English physician Sir William Gull in the mid-1870s later coined the term anorexia nervosa. The symptoms of bulimia (bingeing and purging) were not recognized as a separate condition from self-starvation until the 1940s. English physician Gerald Russell formally named bulimia nervosa in 1979.

At first glance, eating disorders appear to center on worries about food and weight; however, mental health professionals believe these disorders are often about more than simply food. Besides psychological factors that may predispose people to eating disorders, including low self-esteem, depression, anxiety, or loneliness, other factors such as troubled family and personal relationships; difficulty expressing emotions; a history of physical or sexual abuse; or the experience of being teased, taunted, or ridiculed about body size, shape, or weight may increase the risk of developing an eating disorder. Twin and family studies suggest that the tendency to develop an eating disorder also has a genetic origin.

People suffering from eating disorders battle life-threatening obsessions with food and unhealthy thoughts about their body weight and shape. People with the most severe eating disorders are also more likely to have symptoms of depression and low self-esteem. Untreated, these disorders can lead to death. Recovery from an eating disorder is possible, though it is a difficult process that should not be done alone. The first steps toward recovery are for the sufferer to accept that there is a problem and to show a willingness to focus on his or her feelings rather than on food and weight.

Anorexia Nervosa Anorexia nervosa is a condition in which a person refuses to maintain a healthy body weight (persons whose weight is at least 15 percent below their normal body weight fall into this category). Anorexic people starve themselves, even though they may be very hungry. They become terrified of gaining weight and obsessed with food and weight. They often develop strange eating habits, refuse to eat with other people, and exercise strenuously to burn calories and prevent weight gain. People with anorexia continue to believe they are overweight even when they are dangerously thin.

This condition often begins when a girl or young woman who is slightly overweight or normal weight starts to diet to lose weight. After losing weight she wanted to lose, she continues her efforts to lose weight, and dieting becomes an obsession. People with anorexia take pleasure in how well they can avoid eating and measure their self-worth by their ability to lose weight. Eating and weight gain are viewed as weaknesses and personal failures.

In addition to avoiding eating whenever possible, anorexics will often display high levels of energy that seem at odds with their frail physical conditions. They may also develop odd oral habits, including chewing gum throughout the day, drinking an excessive amount of coffee or diet soda, and chain-smoking.

The medical complications of anorexia are similar to starvation. When the body attempts to protect its most vital organs, the heart and the brain, it goes into "slow gear." Menstrual periods stop, and breathing, pulse, blood pressure, and thyroid function slow down. The nails and hair become brittle, the skin dries, and the lack of body fat produces an inability to withstand cold temperatures. In addition, personality changes may occur. The person suffering from anorexia may have outbursts of anger and hostility or may withdraw socially. In the most serious cases, death can result.

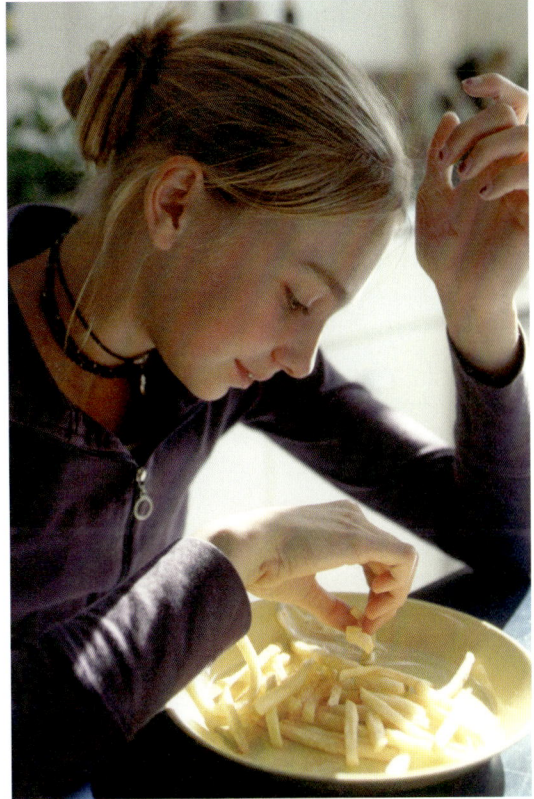

Eating a plate full of French fries is something most teens do occasionally. However, if there is a repeated cycle of binge eating followed by purging, the teen is suffering from bulimia. Such disorders are often difficult to diagnose and treat because of the secretive nature of the illnesses. © DENISE HAGER/ CATCHLIGHT VISUAL SERVICES/ ALAMY.

Bulimia Nervosa People who suffer from bulimia eat compulsively and then purge (get rid of the food) through self-induced vomiting, use of laxatives (drugs that induce bowel movements), diuretics (drugs that expel water from the body through urination), enemas (a process that expels waste from the body by injecting liquid into the anus), strict diets, fasts, exercise, or a combination of several of these compensatory behaviors. Bulimia often begins when a person is disgusted with the excessive amount of food consumed and vomits to get rid of the food and calories.

Many bulimics are at a normal, healthy body weight or above because of their frequent binge-purge behavior, which can occur from once or twice a week to several times per day. Many bulimics who maintain normal weight may manage to keep their eating disorder a secret for years. As with anorexia, bulimia usually begins during adolescence or young adulthood.

A particularly stressful event or depression often triggers an episode of binge eating. The binge eating may temporarily relieve

Eating Disorders Statistics

Eating disorder statistics are estimates because the illnesses are often hidden and difficult to diagnose. It is likely that the actual numbers are higher than they appear because of the secretive nature of eating disorders and sufferers' reluctance to admit that they have a problem. The Eating Disorders Coalition for Research, Policy, and Action reports that:

- About 11 million people in the United States suffer from an eating disorder.

- Anorexia is the third most common illness among adolescents.

- Eating disorders are increasing in younger age groups and are becoming more common in diverse ethnic and sociocultural groups.

- Eating disorders have been diagnosed in children as young as seven years old, 40 percent of nine-year-old girls have dieted, and even five-year-old girls express concern about weight.

- About 40 percent to 60 percent of high school age girls diet, and 13 percent engage in purging.

- About 15 percent of women will suffer from an eating disorder during their lifetime.

a bulimic's feelings of depression or stress, but often deeper feelings of depression, disappointment, and anxiety will follow, which in turn triggers an episode of purging. Many bulimics report feeling out of control when bingeing and use similar terms to describe their need to purge their bodies of the food they just consumed.

Binge eating and purging are dangerous. Purging can result in life-threatening heart conditions because the body loses vital minerals. The acid in vomit wears down tooth enamel and the lining of the esophagus, throat, and mouth and can cause scarring on the hands when fingers are pushed down the throat to induce vomiting.

Many bulimics suffer from low self-esteem and may even have suicidal thoughts. Often they are rigid perfectionists who think in absolutes ("I am bad because I ate that"). Like anorexics, bulimics will make negative statements about their bodies and suffer extreme guilt after eating even normal portions of food. They may begin to withdraw from social activities, particularly those that will make it difficult for them to purge without suspicion.

Binge-Eating Disorder. Binge eating is a common problem among people who are overweight and obese. Besides consuming unusually large amounts of food in a single sitting, binge eaters generally suffer from low mood and low alertness and experience uncontrollable compulsions to eat. They have food cravings before binge episodes and feelings of dissatisfaction and restlessness after binges.

The National Institute of Mental Health (NIMH is one of the National Institutes of Health) reports that binge-eating disorder is the most common eating disorder. Nearly 3% of adults will have a binge-eating disorder at some point in their life.

People who suffer from binge eating often:

- Feel that eating is out of their ability to control
- Eat amounts of food most people would think are unusually large
- Eat much more quickly than usual during binge episodes
- Eat until the point of physical discomfort
- Consume large amounts of food, even when they are not hungry
- Eat alone because they feel embarrassed about the amount of food they eat
- Feel disgusted, depressed, or guilty after overeating

Binge eaters usually suffer from obesity (extreme overweight). Many have been "yo-yo" dieters (experiencing large ups and downs in weight from a cycle of dieting) their entire lives.

Other Types of Disordered Eating There are those eating disorders that do not fall under the categories of anorexia or bulimia; rather, these people exhibit a wide range of disordered eating and unhealthy weight management strategies. Since they cannot be diagnosed as anorexic or bulimic, these individuals will typically receive a diagnosis of an "eating disorder not otherwise specified (EDNOS)." An example of disordered eating is a person of normal weight who eats no fat and occasionally purges. She would not be considered bulimic because she is not bingeing, and she also is not anorexic because she is not dangerously underweight. She would therefore be diagnosed with EDNOS.

Causes of Eating Disorders

Many factors contribute to the development of eating disorders. Some are biological and genetic, while others are a direct result of the cultural and family environments.

Males with Eating Disorders

Although eating disorders affect women more than men, a large number of males suffer from anorexia nervosa and bulimia nervosa as well as binge-eating disorder and exercise addiction. Males account for about 10 percent to 25 percent of people with anorexia or bulimia and about 35 to 40 percent of those with binge-eating disorder. The percentages may even be higher as some experts suspect that few men actually seek help because they are ashamed and embarrassed that they have what has come to be viewed as a "female" problem.

Many male eating-disorder sufferers participate or have participated in a sport that demands a certain body type, such as wrestling and running. Wrestlers are a notoriously high-risk group because many try to lose additional pounds rapidly just prior to a match. This allows the wrestler to compete in a lower weight-class while having developed the skill and strength for a higher weight-class in practice. To accomplish this rapid weight loss, unhealthy weight reduction methods, such as fasting and purging, are often used.

Being overweight in childhood can also influence the development of an eating disorder in males. And dieting, a well-known trigger for eating disorders, can start the development of disordered eating in males just as it may in females.

Biological Factors There are factors contributing to the development of eating disorders that are biological, or genetic. For example, if a person has a relative in her immediate family with an eating disorder, she is at a higher risk to develop an eating disorder.

Disordered eating also may be triggered by the initial act of starving, binge-eating, or purging. This is because these behaviors can change an individual's brain chemistry. Starvation and overeating can both lead to the production of brain chemicals that induce feelings of peace and euphoria (happiness). These good feelings mask feelings of anxiety and depression, both of which are commonly experienced by people suffering from eating disorders. This has caused some researchers to conclude that some people with eating disorders may use food (or starvation) as a way to relieve depression, anxiety, or other emotional upset.

Psychological Factors People suffering from eating disorders share many of the same personality traits. For example, eating-disordered people lean toward being perfectionists. Many of them suffer from low self-esteem, despite their accomplishments and perfectionist ways. Extremist thinking, too, is present in many people with eating disorders. They assume that if being thin is "good" then being even thinner is better. This leads to the thought that being the thinnest is the absolute best; it is this thinking that pushes some anorexics to plummet to body weights of 50 or 60 pounds.

Often, people who live with eating disorders have no sense of self. They simply do not feel that they know who they are or their place in the world. An eating disorder, however, offers a sense of identity to these individuals in that it enables them to say, "I am thin," and "I am dieting." This eventually leads them to define themselves solely on their appearance and their dangerous actions rather than with their positive qualities and accomplishments.

Social Factors Eating disorders, in general, occur primarily in industrialized societies, such as the United States, Australia, Canada, Europe, and Japan. In all of these places, the media (TV, movies, magazines) bombard people with the virtues and importance of being thin. Television, movies, magazines, and advertisements promise that being thin will bring a person success, power, approval, popularity, friends, and romantic relationships. Women, in particular, are held to an almost-impossible-to-achieve standard of physical fitness and beauty, the height of which is being slender and thin. (In fact, female fashion models now weigh an average of 25% less than an average woman.) Because of these media messages, and how young women report feeling about their weight and body shape, a link between eating disorders and social pressures can be established.

Social factors that may contribute to eating disorders include rigid definitions of beauty that exclude people who do not conform to a particular body weight and shape; cultures that glorify thinness and overemphasize the importance of obtaining a "perfect body"; and cultures that judge and value people based on external physical appearance rather than on internal qualities such as character, intellect, generosity, and kindness. Appearance-driven concerns, rather than health needs, continue to motivate many people to lose weight. Society emphasizes these appearance-driven concerns by describing overweight and obese people in a negative manner.

Family Factors People are shaped in part by their experiences with their families. Families contribute to an individual's emotional growth. If someone is raised in a dysfunctional family, he or she may have feelings of abandonment and loneliness. Certain families have dynamics in which rigidity, overprotectiveness, and emotional distance are commonplace. If parents make all of a child's decisions for her, when she becomes a teenager and must make decisions for herself, she may find she doesn't have the tools to do so. All of these dynamics can promote the development of eating disorders in the future.

Families in which unrealistically high expectations are placed on children also may lead people to develop disordered eating. The disordered eating is used as a way to cope with feelings of inadequacy and as a way to control at least one area of their lives.

Children also receive their first messages about their bodies from their families. If parents place too much emphasis on physical appearance, it can lead to low self-esteem in those children, placing them at risk for developing eating disorders when they are older.

Most children learn their eating habits and food preferences from their families. Often times, cleaning one's plate or not eating too much or even parents' close control of the food their children eat can lead to disordered eating later in life. Parents' attitudes toward food and their own bodies greatly affect children's attitudes toward food and how they will feel about themselves.

Famous People who have Battled Eating Disorders

- Paula Abdul, Singer
- Jessica Alba, Actor
- Fiona Apple, Singer and Songwriter
- Justine Bateman, Actor
- Victoria Beckham, Singer and Fashion Designer
- Kate Beckinsale, Actor
- Isabella Caro, Model*
- Karen Carpenter, Singer*
- Kelly Clarkson, Singer
- Nadia Comaneci, Gymnast
- Katie Couric, TV Host
- Portia de Rossi, Actor
- Susan Dey, Actor
- Diana, Princess of Wales
- Calista Flockheart, Actor
- Jane Fonda, Actor/Activist
- Lady Gaga, Singer and Songwriter
- Zina Garrison, Tennis Player
- Tracey Gold, Actor
- Heidi Guenther, Ballet Dancer*
- Lucy Hale, Actor
- Geri Halliwell, Singer
- Margaux Hemingway, Actor
- Christy Henrich, Gymnast*
- Elton John, Musician and Singer

- Daniel Johns, Musician
- Kathy Johnson, Gymnast
- Winona Judd, Singer and Actor
- Gelsey Kirkland, Ballet Dancer
- Lucy Lawless, Actor
- Stacy London, TV Host
- Demi Lovato, Actor and Singer
- Alanis Morissette, Singer
- Mary Kate Olsen, Actor
- Nicole "Snooki" Polizzi, Reality Show Star
- Dennis Quaid, Actor
- Gilda Radner, Actor/Comic
- Tara Reid, Actor
- Nicole Richie, Actor and Designer
- Cathy Rigby, Gymnast
- Joan Rivers, Comic
- Ally Sheedy, Actor
- Ashlee Simpson, Actor and Singer
- Billy Bob Thornton, Actor
- Meredith Viera, TV Host, Anchor, Journalist
- Oprah Winfrey, TV Host, Producer and Actor
- Kate Winslet, Actor

* indicates death resulting from the eating disorder

Triggers Eating disorders are often set off or triggered by an event or a circumstance in the life of an individual who is already prone to developing such a condition. A period of adjustment, such as leaving home to attend summer camp, prep school, or college, can easily trigger disordered eating in an individual with such tendencies already in place. A traumatic event in someone's life, such as sexual abuse, can also trigger the development of an eating disorder. Other triggers may seem harmless yet represent large life changes, such as moving, starting a new school or job, graduation, and even marriage. Triggers are usually closely tied to the end of a valued relationship or a feeling of loneliness.

The most common trigger of an eating disorder, however, is dieting. Very often dieting can lead people to disordered eating of some sort, including anorexia or bulimia.

The Physical and Psychological Consequences of Eating Disorders

An eating disorder can have serious physical and psychological consequences. Untreated, some of the effects of eating disorders are irreversible and life-threatening. For these reasons, early detection and treatment is essential and can save a person's life.

How Anorexia Nervosa Affects the Body Anorexia causes many physical problems. For instance, it upsets the normal functions of hormones. For girls, this means the body is unable to produce enough of the female hormone estrogen because it does not have enough fat. This may cause an absence of menstrual cycles, called amenorrhea. For boys, anorexia causes a decrease in the production of the male hormone testosterone, which results in a loss of sexual interest.

An anorexic body lacks the protective layer of fat it needs to stay warm. To compensate for the lack of fat, lanugo (fine hair) will grow all over the body to keep it warm. Another problem anorexia causes is a decrease in bone mass. The body needs calcium for strong bones. Since an anorexic is not eating enough food, which is the source of calcium, the body's bones suffer and weaken. Later in life, this could

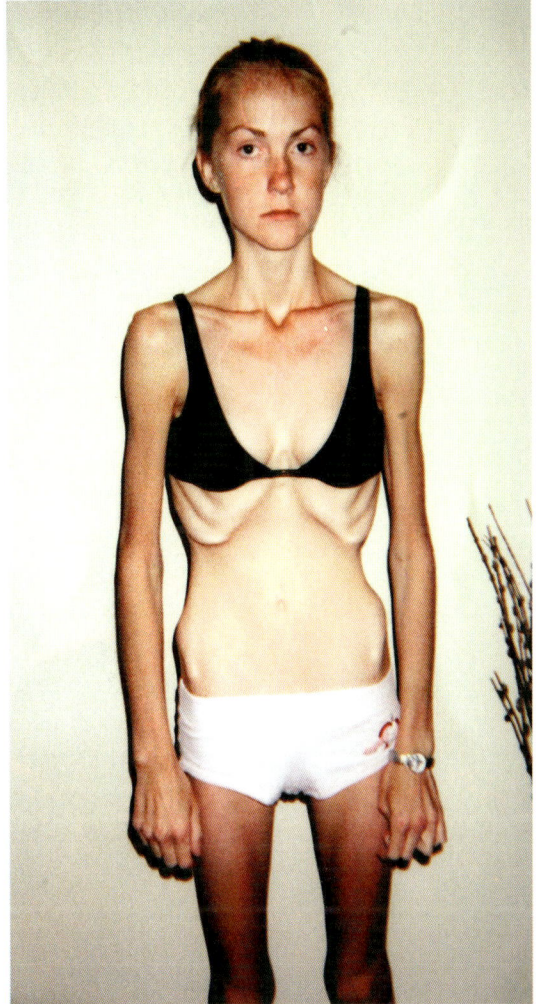

Harriet Smith's decision to eat healthfully at 14 became anorexia. At 5 ft 8 in (1.72 meters) tall, she weighed 70 lbs (31.8 kg) at her thinnest. Even when doctors warned she was so thin her heart could stop, she denied she had a problem. With family support, after a 12 year battle and a year in a specialized treatment unit she was a healthy 133 lbs (60.3 kg). © AP IMAGES/ ALBANPIX LTD/REX FEATURES.

result in dangerously thin, fragile bones—the condition is known as osteoporosis.

Additionally, without the fuel it needs, an anorexic's body will respond as if it is being assaulted and begin to fight back in order to survive. To survive the body must have energy, but because the body has no food to turn into energy, it seeks out the muscles, and eventually, the organs (heart, kidneys, and brain) for sustenance—often causing permanent damage to the organs in the process. This is the most serious consequence of anorexia and can lead to cardiac arrest and/or kidney failure, both of which may result in death.

How Bulimia Nervosa Affects the Body The frequent purging that occurs with bulimia does serious damage to the body. Self-induced vomiting can severely damage the digestive system. Repeated vomiting also damages the esophagus (throat) and eventually it may tear and bleed. Vomiting brings stomach acids into the mouth, causing the enamel on the teeth to wear away. As a result, the teeth may have cavities, become weakened, and appear ragged.

Other consequences include swollen salivary glands, which gives some bulimics the appearance of having chipmunk cheeks, and cuts and sores on the knuckles from repeatedly sticking one's fingers down the throat to induce vomiting (known as "Russell's sign"). Stomach cramps and difficulty in swallowing are also common.

If laxatives (drugs that induce bowel movements) are abused, constipation may result because the body can no longer produce a bowel movement on its own. Abuse of laxatives and diuretics (drugs that expel water from the body through urination) can also cause bloating, water retention, and edema (swelling) of the stomach. Because the body is being denied the nutrients and fluids it needs to survive, the kidneys and heart will also suffer. Specifically, a lack of potassium will result in cardiac abnormalities and possible kidney failure, which may also result in death.

How Binge-Eating Disorder Affects the Body The physical effects of binge eating are not as severe as those of anorexia and bulimia because the body is not denied food or put through the painful process of purging. Nevertheless, there are some potentially serious consequences for binge eaters.

Since binge eaters may suffer from obesity, health complications such as diabetes or heart problems can develop. Health problems from yo-yo dieting can include hypertension (high blood pressure) and long-term damage to major organs, such as the kidneys, liver, heart, and other muscles.

How Exercise Addiction Affects the Body Many anorexics and bulimics exercise compulsively in order to lose weight. Compulsive exercise is extremely dangerous and can cause many painful injuries, including stress fractures, damaged bones and joints, as well as torn muscles, ligaments, and tendons. Even worse, the injuries may become more serious as many compulsive exercisers often continue their routines despite their injuries.

When an eating disorder is successfully treated, the body can heal and return to normal. Sometimes, however, the eating disorder has continued for so many years that there is too much damage for a full recovery to occur. A person may have to live with a weak heart or kidneys for the rest of his or her life. A woman may be unable to conceive a child because her reproductive system cannot function properly or may suffer from the debilitating bone disease osteoporosis.

How Eating Disorders Affect the Mind The psychological consequences of eating disorders are complex and difficult to overcome. An eating disorder is often a symptom of a larger problem in a person's life. The disorder is an unhealthy way to cope with the painful emotions tied to the problem. For this reason, the emotional problems that triggered the eating disorder in the first place can worsen as the disorder takes hold.

Research has shown that many people suffering from an eating disorder also suffer from other psychological problems. Sometimes the eating disorder causes other problems, and sometimes the problems coexist with the eating disorder. Some of the psychological disorders that can accompany an eating disorder include depression, obsessive-compulsive disorder, and anxiety and panic disorders.

In addition to having other psychological disorders, a person with an eating disorder may also engage in destructive behaviors as a result of low self-esteem. Just as an eating disorder is a negative way to cope with emotional problems, other destructive behaviors, such as self-injury and substance abuse, are similar negative coping mechanisms.

Symptoms of Depression

- Extreme mood swings
- Inability to experience pleasure in anything
- Feelings of worthlessness
- Withdrawal from family and friends
- Constant fatigue (exhaustion)
- Insomnia (sleeplessness) or sleeping too much
- Loss of appetite or compulsive eating
- Inability to concentrate or make decisions
- Poor memory
- Unexplained headaches, backaches, or stomachaches

Depression. Depression is one of the most common psychological problems related to an eating disorder. It is characterized by intense and prolonged feelings of sadness and hopelessness. In its most serious form, depression may lead to suicide (the taking of one's own life). Considering that an eating disorder is often a secret, a person who is suffering feels alienated and alone. A person with an eating disorder may feel that it is impossible to openly express his or her feelings. As a result, feelings of depression may worsen the effects of an eating disorder, making it difficult to break the cycle of disordered eating.

With counseling and support, it is possible to combat these negative feelings and prevent them from progressing over time. Psychotherapy, especially cognitive behavioral therapy and other "talk" therapies, can help ease feelings of depression, which in turn gives a person better tools with which to fight an eating disorder.

Obsessive-Compulsive Behavior. Obsessions are constant thoughts that produce anxiety and stress. Compulsions are irrational behaviors that are repeated to reduce anxiety and stress. People with eating disorders are constantly thinking about food, calories, eating, and weight. As a result, they show signs of obsessive-compulsive behavior. When people with eating disorders also show signs of obsessive-compulsive behavior with activities and things not related to food and weight, they may be diagnosed with obsessive-compulsive disorder (OCD).

Some obsessive-compulsive behaviors practiced by eating disorder sufferers include storing large amounts of food, collecting recipes, weighing themselves several times a day, and thinking constantly about the food they feel they should not eat. These obsessive thoughts and rituals worsen when the body is regularly deprived of food. Being in a state of starvation causes people to become so preoccupied with everything they have denied themselves that they think of little else.

Feelings of Anxiety, Guilt, and Shame. Everyone experiences feelings of anxiety (fear and worry), guilt, and shame at some time; however, these

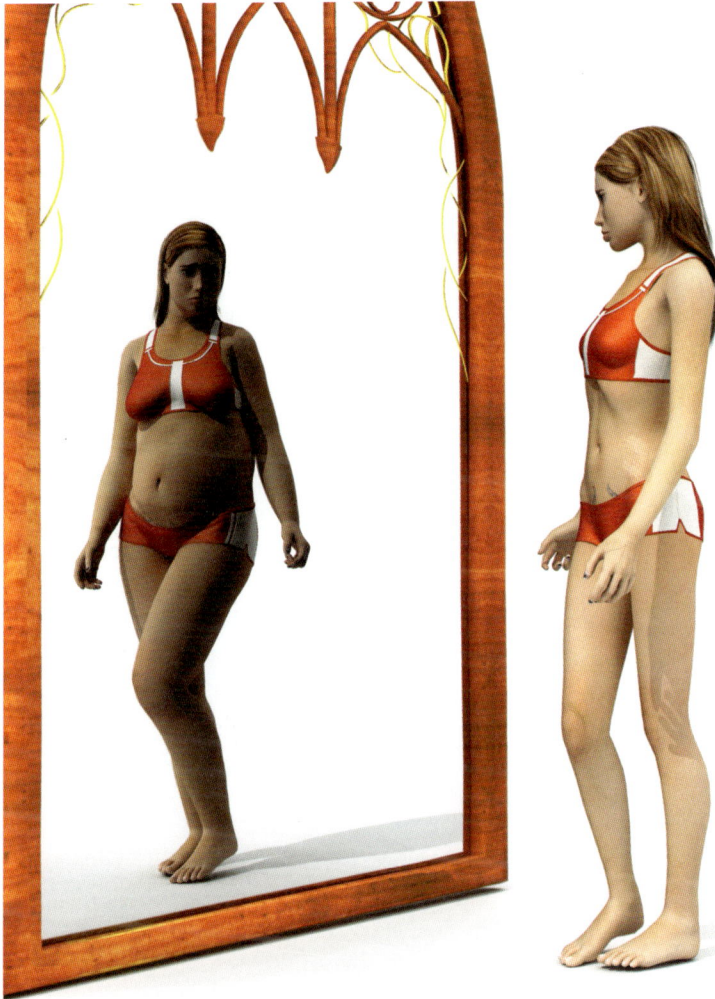

feelings become more intense with the onset of an eating disorder. Eating disorder sufferers fear that others will discover their illness. There is also a tremendous fear of gaining weight.

As the eating disorder progresses, body image becomes more distorted, and the eating disorder becomes all-consuming. Some sufferers are often terrified of letting go of the illness, which causes many to protect their secret eating disorder even more.

Eating disorder sufferers have a strong need to control their environment and will avoid social situations where they may have to be around food in front of other people or where they may have to change their behavior. The anxiety that results causes people with eating disorders to be inflexible and rigid with their emotions.

Bulimics and binge eaters, specifically, experience guilt and shame about their disorders. This is mainly because, unlike anorexics, they are not usually in denial, and they do realize that there is a problem. Bulimics will feel anxiety before, during, and after a binge and can only relieve this anxiety through purging. Purging, however, brings on overwhelming feelings of guilt and shame. Binge eaters also feel anxiety during a binge, but because they do not purge, they feel ashamed over their lack of control around food.

Eating Disorders and Other Destructive Behaviors

Substance Abuse It is common for people with eating disorders also to struggle with drug and/or alcohol addiction. In fact, research shows that one-third of bulimics have a substance-abuse problem, particularly with stimulants (drugs that excite the nervous system) and alcohol. This may stem from the fact that people with eating disorders have difficulty coping with their emotions and use negative means, such as drugs, to mask their problems. Drugs and alcohol provide temporary escapes from reality but, similar to eating disorders, can progress into serious problems that require treatment to overcome.

Eating Disorders and Sexuality

Eating disorders often develop around puberty, when the body is changing and maturing. This time of change can produce anxiety and confusion for both boys and girls because puberty is the beginning of sexual maturity. Girls develop breasts, start menstruating, grow taller, and develop more body hair. Boys' sexual organs (the penis and testicles) grow. Boys also grow taller, get more body and facial hair, and develop bigger muscles.

The sexual feelings that accompany puberty are new, and these feelings may embarrass some young people. When someone is suffering from an eating disorder, issues surrounding sexuality can become even more complicated. Some people may seek out sexual relationships to feel close to someone and ease feelings of isolation. Others may avoid sexual relationships altogether because they feel ashamed of their bodies.

In some cases, an eating disorder is triggered by sexual abuse. In these instances, an eating disorder sufferer is usually acting out in response to a painful event. She may gain or lose weight in an attempt to make herself sexually undesirable. She may avoid sexual relations as a way to take control of her body and prevent painful feelings from resurfacing. The anger and distrust felt toward the opposite sex may result in complete rejection of the opposite sex. On the other hand, some eating disorder sufferers may have many sexual partners in an attempt to erase the past and gain acceptance from the opposite sex.

Treatment and Recovery from Eating Disorders

Treatment and recovery go hand in hand. It is very hard to recover from an eating disorder without any treatment. Recovery is a long process, and some eating disorder sufferers may have to enter treatment more than once. Some people may even try different kinds of treatment programs during their recovery until they find one that works for them.

There may be obstacles to starting treatment. The fear of becoming fat and losing control, which drives most eating disorders, is very strong and hard to eliminate. Also, eating disorder sufferers may be in denial about their condition and may be unwilling to consider treatment. These feelings may be based on a fear of letting go of the illness that they feel is part of their identity. Eating disorder sufferers must learn to refocus their thoughts from food and weight to their emotions so that they can deal with the root cause of the disorder. Since many feelings that need to be addressed have been buried by the disorder, professional counseling is important for a successful recovery.

In order for treatment to work, a person must be ready to be treated. Some sufferers may even say they are ready but really are not. They may pretend to change their attitude about food, but they are still starving

Some Web Sites Promote Dangerous Eating Disorders

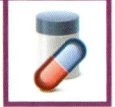

There are many Web sites and Internet resources that can help to inform and support people struggling with eating disorders. Unfortunately, the Internet also has Web sites, known as "Pro-Ana" (pro-anorexia) and "Pro-Mia" (pro-bulimia) that actually promote and encourage eating disordered behaviors.

These Web sites portray eating disorders as lifestyle choices rather than serious illnesses. Many of the Web sites have photos of bone-thin girls and women and offer a variety of unrealistic and unhealthy weight-loss plans, tips to reduce hunger pangs, and other encouragement of eating disordered behaviors. "Thinspiration" is the term these Web sites use for photographs of dangerously thin women that are intended to motivate unhealthy weight loss.

Some of these pro-ED Web sites and social media sites also use forums and chat rooms where people with eating disorders can share ideas and stories about their eating disorders. The danger is that instead of getting support for recovering from their eating disorders, visitors to these Web sites interact with people who support their actions instead of questioning and encouraging them to get needed treatment.

themselves or bingeing and purging their food secretively. When people do not fully commit to a treatment program, they will most likely continue suffering from the deadly illness even after completion of the program.

Treatment Basics Treatment usually begins with an assessment by a physician or mental health counselor. Depending on the severity of the eating disorder, the sufferer will either enter an inpatient or outpatient program. Inpatient programs, or hospitalization, are for the most severe cases. To be hospitalized, the sufferer is usually at a critical point in the illness where his or her life is in danger or at risk because of strong suicidal thoughts. Outpatient programs are conducted at a facility or doctor's office that the patient visits while still living at home.

Whether the program is inpatient or outpatient, it will usually include various forms of counseling and medical care to treat the physical effects of the illness. The most common forms of counseling include nutrition, individual, family, and group. Nutrition counseling teaches the patient about healthy eating habits and designs appropriate meals. Its goal is to slowly bring the sufferer's weight back up to a safe level that can be easily maintained without dieting or provoking obsessive behavior about food.

Cognitive-behavioral therapy (CBT) teaches people how to monitor their eating and change unhealthy eating habits. It also teaches them how to change the way they respond to stressful situations. Interpersonal psychotherapy (IPT) helps people look at their relationships with friends and family and make changes to resolve problems. Group therapy has been found helpful for bulimics, who are relieved to find that they are not alone or unique in their eating behavior.

A combination of behavioral therapy and family systems therapy is often effective with anorexics. Family therapy considers the family as the unit of treatment and focuses on relationships and communication patterns within the family rather than on the personality traits or symptoms displayed by individual family members. Problems are addressed by changing how the family works and responds to problems rather than by trying to change an individual family member. People with eating disorders who also suffer from depression sometimes benefit from medications to help relieve symptoms of depression and anxiety.

Group therapy has been found helpful for bulimics, who are relieved to find that they are not alone or unique in their eating behavior.

In support groups, eating disorder sufferers meet to offer support, understanding, and hope to one another as they battle their disorders. Support groups, like group counseling, help sufferers to not feel so alone in their illnesses and learn from others' experiences.

The Recovery Process Recovery is not easy. With treatment, which can take months to years, about one-third of people with eating disorders recover, one-third vary between recovery and relapse, and the remaining third do not recover. To recover fully, people with eating disorders need to build their self-esteem so that they can believe that they deserve the love of others. Some people are able to make an initial recovery, but many find recovery to be an ongoing, lifelong process.

An eating disorder sufferer has certain goals, both physical and psychological, that he or she needs to try to reach in recovery. The physical aims should include the ability to eat a variety of healthful foods (without bingeing and purging) and maintain a healthy weight. Females should start their menstrual periods either for the first time or again without the help of medication.

The psychological aims of recovery should include a noticeable decrease in the fear of food and becoming fat as well as the ability to establish strong relationships with family and friends again. Another goal is to realize the role society and the media play in furthering disordered thinking about people's weights and body shapes. This realization can help sufferers learn to accept their bodies without having to live up to unrealistic standards of beauty and thinness. An eating disorder sufferer also must learn and practice positive coping skills and engage in activities that do not involve food or weight control.

Preventing Eating Disorders

Many eating disorder organizations focus on prevention—stopping eating disorders before they even start. The belief is that awareness and

What to Do If You Think Someone Has an Eating Disorder

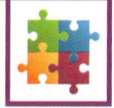

- First, voice concerns to the person privately.
- Listen carefully to what that person is saying.
- Avoid using judgmental statements.
- Let the person know that you are concerned about his or her health.
- Be familiar with some resources, such as reading materials, Web sites, or community centers, that can be introduced to that person.
- If the person exhibits behaviors that are life-threatening, such as bingeing and purging several times a day, fainting, or expressing suicidal thoughts, tell a trusted adult immediately.

education can go a long way in preventing these painful disorders, which can become lifelong struggles. Many eating disorder experts promote teaching prevention at a young age since eating disorders usually begin in adolescence.

Prevention programs aim to provide people with the tools they need to cope with the problems that may contribute to an eating disorder.

Prevention means:

- reordering thoughts on food and weight
- focusing on health
- understanding the dangers of dieting
- developing a positive body image
- rebelling against cultural and media messages that encourage unhealthy behaviors
- explaining why fat is not the enemy
- helping to end fat discrimination

Media images that create, reflect, communicate, and reinforce cultural definitions of attractiveness, especially for girls and women, are factors that contribute to the rise of eating disorders. They exert powerful influences on values, attitudes, and practices for body image, diet, and activity. When they promote unrealistic standards of female beauty and unhealthy eating habits, they contribute to the growing problem of eating disorders.

Reordering Thoughts about Food and Weight The first step in preventing the development of eating disorders is to reorder feelings and thoughts about food and weight. Eating disorder experts recommend that people reject unhealthy messages about weight, body shape, and diet. Since body shape and weight are determined mostly by genetics, there is only so much a person can do to control or change weight and body shape. Trying to fight against or change the body's set point (the weight at which one's body naturally falls) is unhealthy and possibly dangerous because it creates a cycle of yo-yo dieting. Research has shown that while not every diet leads to eating disorders, 80 percent of eating disorders are initially triggered by dieting.

Developing a Positive Body Image

Developing a positive body image is necessary to the prevention of eating disorders. Many people struggle with this issue and must work hard at accepting their bodies. Eating disorder experts emphasize the importance of exercising for health reasons rather than to burn calories and lose weight. The same experts also recommend becoming politically active in the fight against unhealthy cultural messages because this fight can be a source of positive feelings and empowerment.

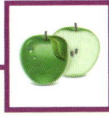

How Does Dieting Affect the Body and Mind?

The body needs a certain amount of food to function properly. If caloric intake is restricted and the body falls below its set point, it will respond by lowering its metabolism. Metabolism is the rate at which the body burns energy. When the body doesn't get enough fuel to burn, it must learn to function on less. In response, the body will hold on to any food it gets and store fat more efficiently on fewer calories. Typically, when people stop dieting, they gain more weight than they lost and are likely to keep the extra weight because the body has made adjustments to compensate for a lack of food from the dieting.

The negative physical effects of dieting can include:

- headaches
- dizziness
- stomach pain

- iron deficiency that causes fatigue
- possible menstrual irregularity
- lack of estrogen
- calcium deficiency
- lack of growth from malnutrition

The negative psychological effects of dieting can include:

- preoccupation with food, eating, and calories
- increased irritability
- increased stress and anxiety from semi-starvation
- inability to determine hunger and fullness
- negative body image that can lead to depression and low self-esteem
- fear of food that can lead to isolation and alienation

Other suggestions include:

- Avoid negative talk about food and weight.
- Avoid referring to foods as "good" or "bad."
- Don't participate in weight-loss programs or experiment with weight-loss products.
- Exercise moderately; don't engage in unhealthy or excessive exercise programs.
- Talk about body-image issues with close friends and family.
- Don't criticize people for gaining weight.
- Don't compliment people for losing weight.
- Encourage family and friends to question societal and cultural attitudes about weight and body shape.

For More Information

BOOKS

Arnold, Carrie, and B. Timothy Walsh. *Next to Nothing: A Firsthand Account of One Teenager's Experience with an Eating Disorder.* New York: Oxford University Press, 2007.

Covey, Sean. *The 6 Most Important Decisions You'll Ever Make: A Guide for Teens.* New York: Touchstone, 2006.

KidsPeace, and Martha Radev, ed. *I've Got This Friend Who: Advice for Teens and Their Friends on Alcohol, Drugs, Eating Disorders, Risky Behavior and More.* Center City, MN: Hazelden, 2007.

Magill, Elizabeth, ed. *Drug Information for Teens: Health Tips about the Physical and Mental Effects of Substance Abuse Including Information about Alcohol, Tobacco, Marijuana, Prescription and Over-the-counter Drugs, Club Drugs, Hallucinogens, Stimulants, Opiates, Steroids, and More*, 3rd ed. Detroit, MI: Omnigraphics, 2011.

Nelson, Tammy. *What's Eating You?: A Workbook for Teens with Anorexia, Bulimia, and Other Eating Disorders.* Oakland, CA: Instant Help/New Harbinger Publications, 2008.

Schulherr, Susan. *Eating Disorders For Dummies.* Hoboken, NJ: Wiley, 2008.

Shapiro, Lawrence E. *Stopping the Pain: A Workbook for Teens Who Cut and Self Injure.* Oakland, CA: Instant Help Books, 2008.

WEB SITES

The Alliance for Eating Disorders Awareness. http://www.allianceforeatingdisorders.com (accessed December 27, 2012).

"Cause: Physical and Mental Health: Body Image." *DoSomething.org.* http://www.dosomething.org/cause/physical-and-mental-health (accessed November 12, 2012).

"Cause: Physical and Mental Health: Drug Abuse." *DoSomething.org.* http://www.dosomething.org/cause/physical-and-mental-health (accessed November 12, 2012).

"Eating Disorders." *National Institute of Mental Health.* http://www.nimh.nih.gov/health/topics/eating-disorders/index.shtml (accessed December 27, 2012).

National Eating Disorders Association. http://www.nationaleatingdisorders.org/ (accessed December 27, 2012).

The Nemours Foundation. "TeensHealth: Drugs & Alcohol." *KidsHealth.org.* http://kidshealth.org/teen/drug_alcohol/ (accessed November 22, 2012).

The Nemours Foundation. "TeensHealth: Eating Disorders." *KidsHealth.org.* http://kidshealth.org/teen/food_fitness/problems/eat_disorder.html#cat20135 (accessed November 22, 2012).

The Nemours Foundation. "TeensHealth: Prescription Drug Abuse." *KidsHealth.org.* http://kidshealth.org/teen/drug_alcohol/drugs/prescription_drug_abuse.html (accessed November 22, 2012).

"NIDA for Teens: The Science Behind Drug Abuse" *National Institutes of Health: National Institute on Drug Abuse.* http://www.teens.drugabuse.gov (accessed December 27, 2012).

The Partnership at DrugFree.org. http://www.drugfree.org (accessed December 27, 2012).

"The Science of Drug Abuse & Addiction." *National Institutes of Health: National Institute on Drug Abuse.* http://www.drugabuse.gov (accessed December 27, 2012).

"The Science of Drug Abuse & Addiction: Students and Young Adults." *National Institutes of Health: National Institute on Drug Abuse.* http://www.drugabuse.gov/students-young-adults (accessed December 27, 2012).

Substance Abuse and Mental Health Services Administration. http://www.samhsa.gov (accessed December 27, 2012).

List of Organizations

The Alliance for Eating Disorders Awareness

P.O. Box 2562
West Palm Beach, FL 33402
USA
Phone: (866) 662-1235
E-mail: info@eatingdisorderinfo.org
Internet: http://www.allianceforeating disorders.com

The American Academy of Child and Adolescent Psychiatry

3615 Wisconsin Avenue, NW
Washington, DC 20016-3007
USA
Phone: (202) 966-7300
Fax: (202) 966-2891
Internet: http://www.aacap.org

American Association of Poison Control Centers

515 King St., Suite 510
Alexandria, Virginia 22314
USA
Phone: (800) 222-1222
Fax: (703) 894-1858
E-mail: info@aapcc.org
Internet: http://www.aapcc.org/

American Medical Association

515 N. State Street
Chicago, IL 60654
USA
Phone: (800) 621-8335
Internet: http://www.ama-assn.org/ama/pub/patients/patients.page

American Psychiatric Association

1000 Wilson Boulevard, Suite 1825
Arlington, VA 22209
USA
Phone: (888) 357-7924
E-mail: apa@psych.org
Internet: http://www.psych.org

American Psychological Association

750 First Street, NE
Washington, DC 20002-4242
USA
Phone: (800) 374-2721
Internet: http://www.apa.org/

American Yoga Association

P.O. Box 19986
Sarasota, FL 34276
USA
E-mail: info@americanyogaassociation.org
Internet: http://www.americanyogaassociation.org/contents.html

Centers for Disease Control and Prevention
1600 Clifton Rd.
Atlanta, GA 30333
USA
Phone: (800) 232-4636
Internet: http://www.cdc.gov/

Children's Environmental Health Network
110 Maryland Avenue NE, Suite 402
Washington, DC 20002
USA
Phone: (202) 543-4033
Fax: (202) 543-8797
E-mail: cehn@cehn.org
Internet: http://www.cehn.org

Earth Force
2555 W. 34th Avenue
Denver, CO 80211
USA
Phone: (303) 433-2956
Fax: (888) 899-5324
E-mail: earthforce@earthforce.org
Internet: http://www.earthforce.org/

Environmental Health Coalition
2727 Hoover Ave., Suite 202
National City, CA 91950
USA
Phone: (619) 474-0220
Fax: (619) 474-1210
E-mail: ehc@environmentalhealth.org
Internet: http://www.environmentalhealth.org

Families USA
1201 New York Avenue NW, Suite 1100
Washington, DC 20005
USA
Phone: (202) 628-3030
Fax: (202) 347-2417
E-mail: info@familiesusa.org
Internet: http://www.familiesusa.org/

Food and Water Watch
1616 P St. NW, Suite 300
Washington, DC 20036
USA
Phone: (202) 683-2500
E-mail: foodandwater@fwwatch.org
Internet: http://foodandwaterwatch.org/

Gay & Lesbian Advocates & Defenders (GLAAD)
5455 Wilshire Blvd, Number 1500
Los Angeles, CA 90036
USA
Phone: (323) 933-2240
Fax: (323) 933-2241
Internet: http://www.glaad.org/

Healthy Child Healthy World
12300 Wilshire Blvd., Suite 320
Los Angeles, CA 90025
USA
Phone: (310) 820-2030
Fax: (310) 820-2070
Internet: http://www.healthychild.org

National Alliance on Mental Illness
3803 N. Fairfax Dr., Suite 100
Arlington, VA 22203
USA
Phone: (703) 524-7600
Phone: (800) 950-6264
Fax: (703) 524-9094
Internet: http://www.nami.org/

National Eating Disorders Association
165 West 46th Street
New York, NY 10036
USA
Phone: (800) 931-2237 (helpline)
Phone: (212) 575-6200
Fax: (212) 575-1650
E-mail: info@NationalEatingDisorders.org
Internet: http://www.nationaleatingdisorders.org/

The Partnership at Drugfree.org

352 Park Avenue South, 9th Floor
New York, NY 10010
USA
Phone: (212) 922-1560
Phone: (855) 378-4373 (helpline)
Fax: (212) 922-1570
E-mail: webmail@drugfree.org
Internet: http://www.drugfree.org/

Planned Parenthood

434 West 33rd Street
New York, NY 10001
USA
Phone: (212) 541-7800
Phone: (800) 230-7526
Fax: (212) 245-1845
Internet: http://www.plannedparenthood.org/

President's Council on Fitness, Sports & Nutrition

1101 Wootton Parkway, Suite 560
Rockville, MD 20852
USA
Phone: (240) 276-9567
Fax: (240) 276-9860
E-mail: fitness@hhs.gov
Internet: http://www.fitness.gov/

Rape, Abuse, and Incest National Network

2000 L Street NW, Suite 406
Washington, DC 20036
USA
Phone: (800) 656-4673 (helpline)
Phone: (202) 544-1034
Fax: (202) 544-3556
E-mail: info@rainn.org
Internet: http://centers.rainn.org/

Rudd Center for Food Policy and Obesity

P.O. Box 208369
New Haven, CT 06520
USA

Phone: (203) 432-6700
Internet: http://www.yaleruddcenter.org

School Nutrition Association

700 S. Washington St., Suite 300
Alexandria, VA 22314
USA
Phone: (703) 739-3900
Fax: (703) 739-3915
E-mail: servicecenter@schoolnutrition.org
Internet: http://www.schoolnutrition.org

U.S. Environmental Protection Agency (EPA)

Ariel Rios Building
1200 Pennsylvania Avenue, NW
Washington, DC 20460
USA
Phone: (202) 272-0167
Internet: http://www.epa.gov

U.S. Department of Agriculture (USDA)

1400 Independence Avenue, SW
Washington, DC 20250
USA
Phone: (202) 720-2791
Internet: http://www.usda.gov

U.S. Food and Drug Administration (FDA)

10903 New Hampshire Avenue
Silver Spring, MD 20993
USA
Phone: (888) 463-6332
Internet: http://www.fda.gov/

U.S. National Human Genome Research Institute

Building 31, Room 4B09
31 Center Drive, MSC 2152
9000 Rockville Pike
Bethesda, MD 20892-2152
USA
Phone: (301) 402-0911
Fax: (301) 402-2218
Internet: http://www.genome.gov/

U.S. National Institute of Mental Health (NIMH)

6001 Executive Boulevard,
Room 6200, MSC 9663
Bethesda, MD 20892
USA
Phone: (866) 615-6464
Fax: (301) 443-4279
E-mail: nimhinfo@nih.gov
Internet: http://www.nimh.nih.gov

U.S. National Institute on Drug Abuse (NIDA)

6001 Executive Boulevard,
Room 5213, MSC 9561
Bethesda, MD 20892-9561
USA
Phone: (301) 443-1124
E-mail: information@nida.nih.gov
Internet: http://www.drugabuse.gov/

U.S. National Institutes of Health (NIH)

9000 Rockville Pike
Bethesda, MD 20892
USA
Phone: (301) 496-4000
E-mail: NIHinfo@od.nih.gov
Internet: http://nih.gov/

U.S. Substance Abuse and Mental Health Services Administration (SAMHSA)

1 Choke Cherry Road
Rockville, MD 20857
USA
Phone: (877) 726-4727
E-mail: SAMHSAInfo@samhsa.hhs.gov
Internet: http://www.samhsa.gov

The Vegetarian Resource Group

P.O. Box 1463
Baltimore, MD 21203
USA
Phone: (410) 366-8343
E-mail: vrg@vrg.org
Internet: http://www.vrg.org/

Yum-O Organization

132 E. 43rd St., No. 223
New York, NY 10017
USA
Phone: (410) 366-8343
E-mail: info@yum-o.org
Internet: http://www.yum-o.org/

Where to Learn More

Books

American Medical Association. *American Medical Association Girl's Guide to Becoming a Teen.* San Francisco: Jossey-Bass, 2006.

Andrews, John. *Dare To Make A Difference—Success 101 For Teens.* New York: BTWEYL, 2010.

Arnold, Carrie, and B. Timothy Walsh. *Next to Nothing: A Firsthand Account of One Teenager's Experience with an Eating Disorder.* New York: Oxford University Press, 2007.

Bailey, Jacqui. *Sex, Puberty, and All That Stuff: A Guide to Growing Up.* New York: Barron's, 2004.

Bakewell, Lisa, ed. *Fitness Information for Teens: Health Tips About Exercise, Physical Well-being, and Health Maintenance (Teen Health Series).* Toronto: Omnigraphics Inc, 2008.

Barondes, Samuel. *Making Sense of People: Decoding the Mysteries of Personality.* Upper Saddle River, NJ: FT Press, 2012.

Belliner, Karen, and Zachary Klimecki, eds. *Sports Injuries Information for Teens.* Detroit, MI: Omnigraphics, 2012.

Bijlefeld, Marjolijn, and Sharon Zoumbaris. *Food and You: A Guide to Healthy Habits for Teens.* Westport: Greenwood, 2001.

The Boston Women's Health Collective. *Our Bodies, Ourselves*, 40th Anniversary Rev. ed. New York: Touchstone, 2011.

Bowden, Jonny. *The Most Effective Natural Cures on Earth: The Surprising, Unbiased Truth about What Treatments Work and Why.* BC, Canada: Fair Winds Press, 2011.

Capacchione, Lucia. *The Art of Emotional Healing.* Boston: Shambhala, 2006.

Capacchione, Lucia. *The Creative Journal for Teens: Making Friends with Yourself*, 2nd ed. Franklin Lakes, NJ: New Page Books, 2002.

Carlseon, Dale. *The Teen Brain Book: Who and What Are You?* Madison, CT: Bick Publishing House, 2004.

Carson, Rachel. *Silent Spring*, 40th Anniversary ed. New York: Houghton Mifflin Company, 2002.

Ciarrochi, Joseph, Louise Hayes, and Ann Bailey. *Get Out of Your Mind and Into Your Life for Teens: A Guide to Living an Extraordinary Life.* Oakland, CA: Instant Help, 2012.

Cooper, Barbara, and Nancy Widdows. *The Social Success Workbook for Teens: Skill-Building Activities for Teens with Nonverbal Learning Disorder, Asperger's Disorder, and Other Social-Skill Problems.* Oakland, CA: Instant Help, 2008.

Covey, Sean. *The 6 Most Important Decisions You'll Ever Make: A Guide for Teens.* New York: Touchstone, 2006.

Crump, Marguerite. *No B.O.!: The Head-to-Toe Book of Hygiene for Preteens.* New York: Free Spirit Publishing, 2002.

Dawson, Peg, and Richard Guare. *Smart but Scattered: The Revolutionary "Executive Skills" Approach to Helping Kids Reach Their Potential.* New York: Guilford Press, 2013.

Dunham, Kelli. *The Boy's Body Book: Everything You Need to Know for Growing Up YOU.* New York: Applesauce Press, 2007.

Dunham, Kelli. *The Girl's Body Book: Everything You Need to Know for Growing Up YOU.* New York: Applesauce Press, 2008.

Faigenbaum, Avery, and Wayne Westcott. *Youth Strength Training.* Champaign, IL: Human Kinetics, 2009.

Ford, Emily, Michael Liebowitz, and Linda Wasmer Andrews. *What You Must Think of Me: A Firsthand Account of One Teenager's Experience with Social Anxiety Disorder.* New York: New York: Oxford University Press, 2007.

Fox, Marci, and Leslie Sokol. *Think Confident, Be Confident for Teens: A Cognitive Therapy Guide to Overcoming Self-Doubt and Creating Unshakable Self-Esteem.* Oakland, CA: Instant Help Books, 2011.

Furgang, Kathy. *Frequently Asked Questions about Sports Injuries.* New York: Rosen Publishing Group, 2007.

Gaede, Katrina, Alan Lachica, and Doug Werner. *Fitness Training for Girls: A Teen Girl's Guide to Resistance Training, Cardiovascular Conditioning and Nutrition.* Cambridgeshire: Tracks Publishing, 2001.

Garofalo, Rob. *A Winner by Any Standard: A Personal Growth Journey for Every American Teen.* New York: Teen Winners Publishing, 2004.

Gay, Kathlyn. *Living Green: The Ultimate Teen Guide (It Happened to Me).* New York: Scarecrow Press, 2012.

Gold, Rozanne, and Phil Mansfield. *Eat Fresh Food: Awesome Recipes for Teen Chefs.* New York: Bloomsbury USA Childrens, 2009.

Harris, Robie. *It's Perfectly Normal: Changing Bodies, Growing Up, Sex, and Sexual Health.* New York: Candlewick, 2009.

Hasan, Heather. *Frequently Asked Questions about Everyday First Aid.* New York: Rosen Publishing Group, 2009.

Hawkins, Frank C. *The Boy's Fitness Guide*. Boy's Guide Book, 2008.

Hicks, Angela. *The Acupuncture Handbook: How Acupuncture Works and How It Can Help You*. London, UK: Piatkus Books, 2011.

Hutchins Paquette, Penny, and Cheryl Gerson Tuttle. *Learning Disabilities: The Ultimate Teen Guide (It Happened to Me)*. Lanham, MD: Scarecrow Press, 2006.

Hyde, Margaret O. *Drugs 101: An Overview for Teens*. Brookfield, CT: Twenty-First Century Books, 2003.

Jamieson, Patrick E., and Moira A. Rynn. *Mind Race: A Firsthand Account of One Teenager's Experience with Bipolar Disorder*. New York: Oxford University Press, 2006.

Kaye, Cathryn Berger, and Philippe Cousteau. *Going Blue: A Teen Guide to Saving Our Oceans, Lakes, Rivers, & Wetlands*. Minneapolis, MN: Free Spirit, 2010.

Kellerman, Henry. *Personality: How It Forms*. New York: American Mental Health Foundation Books, 2012.

KidsPeace, and Martha Radev, ed. *I've Got this Friend Who: Advice for Teens and Their Friends on Alcohol, Drugs, Eating Disorders, Risky Behaviors, and More*. Center City, MN: Hazelden, 2007.

Lawrience, Michael. *Self-Esteem: A Teen's Guide for Girls*. Lawrience Publishing, 2012.

Locricchio, Matthew. *Teen Cuisine*. New York: Marshall Cavendish, 2010.

Locricchio, Matthew. *Teen Cuisine: New Vegetarian*. New York: Marshall Cavendish Children, 2012.

Madaras, Lynda. *What's Happening to My Body? Book for Boys.*, Rev. ed. New York: William Morrow Paperbacks, 2007.

Madaras, Lynda. *What's Happening to My Body? Book for Girls*, Rev. ed. New York: William Morrow Paperbacks, 2007.

Madison, Lynda. *The Feelings Book: The Care & Keeping of Your Emotions*. Wisconsin: American Girl, 2002.

Magill, Elizabeth, ed. *Drug Information for Teens: Health Tips about the Physical and Mental Effects of Substance Abuse Including Information about Alcohol, Tobacco, Marijuana, Prescription and Over-the-counter Drugs, Club Drugs, Hallucinogens, Stimulants, Opiates, Steroids, and More*, 3rd ed. Detroit, MI: Omnigraphics, 2011.

Mar, Jonathan, and Grace Norwich. *The Body Book for Boys*. New York: Scholastic, 2010.

Mayo Clinic. *Mayo Clinic Book of Alternative Medicine: Integrating the Best Natural Therapies with Conventional Medicine*, 2nd ed. New York: Oxmoor House, 2010.

McCoy, Kathy, and Charles Wibbelsman. *The Teenage Body Book*, Rev. and updated ed. New York: Hatherleigh Press, 2008.

McDuffie, Lora. *Hygiene & Appearance: What Every Pre-teen and Teenage Girl Should Know*. New York: PublishAmerica, 2009.

Mindell, Earl, and Virginia Hopkins. *Prescription Alternatives: Safe, Natural, Prescription-Free Remedies to Restore and Maintain Your Health*, 4th ed. New York: McGraw-Hill, 2009.

Murray, Michael, and Joseph Pizzorno. *The Encyclopedia of Natural Medicine*, 3rd ed. New York: Atria Books, 2012.

Nelson, Tammy. *What's Eating You?: A Workbook for Teens with Anorexia, Bulimia, and Other Eating Disorders.* Oakland, CA: Instant Help/New Harbinger Publications, 2008.

Nettle, Daniel. *Personality: What Makes You the Way You Are.* New York: Oxford University Press, USA, 2009.

Palmer, Pat, and Melissa Alberti Froehner. *Teen Esteem: A Self-Direction Manual for Young Adults.* Atascadero, CA: Impact Publishers, Inc., 2010.

Pampel, Fred C. *Prescription Drugs.* New York: Facts On File, 2010.

Purperhart, Helen. *Yoga Exercises for Teens: Developing a Calmer Mind and a Stronger Body.* Alameda, CA: Hunter House Publishers, 2009.

Roizen, Michael F., and Mehmet C. Oz. *YOU: The Owner's Manual for Teens: A Guide to a Healthy Body and Happy Life.* New York: Free Press, 2011.

Sayler, Mary Harwell. *Prescription Pain Relievers.* New York: Chelsea House, 2011.

Schab, Lisa M. *Beyond the Blues: A Workbook to Help Teens Overcome Depression.* Oakland, CA: Instant Help Books, 2008.

Schab, Lisa M. *The Anxiety Workbook for Teens.* Oakland, CA: Instant Help Books, 2008.

Scheckel, Larry. *Ask Your Science Teacher: Answers to Everyday Questions: Things You Always Wanted to Know about How the World Works.* CreateSpace Independent Publishing Platform, 2011.

Schiraldi, Glenn. *The Self-Esteem Workbook.* Oakland, CA: New Harbinger Publications, 2001.

Schulherr, Susan. *Eating Disorders For Dummies.* Hoboken, NJ: Wiley, 2008.

Shanley, Ellen, and Colleen Thompson. *Fueling the Teen Machine.* Boulder: Bull Publishing Company, 2010.

Shapiro, Lawrence E. *Stopping the Pain: A Workbook for Teens Who Cut and Self Injure.* Oakland, CA: Instant Help Books, 2008.

Sivertsen, Linda, and Tosh Sivertsen. *Generation Green: The Ultimate Teen Guide to Living an Eco-Friendly Life.* New York: Simon Pulse, 2008.

Stille, Darlene. *Genetics: A Living Blueprint.* Minnesota: Compass Point Books, 2006.

Taudte, Jeca, and Dan Santat. *MySpace/OurPlanet: Change Is Possible.* New York: HarperCollins, 2008.

Tuttle, Cheryl Gerson. *Medications: The Ultimate Teen Guide.* Lanham, MD: Scarecrow Press, 2005.

Van Dijk, Sheri. *Don't Let Your Emotions Run Your Life for Teens: Dialectical Behavior Therapy Skills for Helping You Manage Mood Swings, Control Angry Outbursts, and Get Along with Others.* Oakland, CA: Instant Help Books, 2011.

Wood, Jeffrey C. *Getting Help: The Complete & Authoritative Guide to Self-Assessment and Treatment of Mental Health Problems.* Oakland, CA: New Harbinger Publications, 2007.

Zelinger, Laurie, and Jennifer Kalis. *A Smart Girl's Guide to Liking Herself, Even on the Bad Days.* Middleton, WI: American Girl, 2012.

Web Sites

The Alliance for Eating Disorders Awareness. http://www.allianceforeatingdisorders.com (accessed December 27, 2012).

American Academy of Child and Adolescent Psychiatry. http://www.aacap.org (accessed December 11, 2012).

American Academy of Physician Assistants. http://www.aapa.org (accessed November 29, 2012).

American Art Therapy Association. http://www.arttherapy.org (accessed November 28, 2012).

American Association of Colleges of Pharmacy. http://www.aacp.org (accessed November 28, 2012).

American Association of Naturopathic Physicians. http://www.naturopathic.org (accessed November 28, 2012).

American Association of Poison Control Centers (AAPCC). http://www.aapcc.org/. Emergency Poisoning Hotline: 800-222-1222. (accessed November 19, 2012).

American Chiropractic Association. http://www.amerchiro.org (accessed November 28, 2012).

American Counseling Association. http://www.counseling.org (accessed November 28, 2012).

American Dental Association. http://www.ada.org (accessed November 28, 2012).

The American Foundation for AIDS Research. http://amfar.org (accessed November 8, 2012).

American Massage Therapy Association. http://www.amtamassage.org (accessed November 28, 2012).

American Medical Association. http://www.ama-assn.org (accessed November 28, 2012).

American Nurses Association. http://www.nursingworld.org (accessed November 28, 2012).

American Occupational Therapy Association. http://www.aota.org (accessed November 28, 2012).

American Optometric Association. http://www.aoa.org (accessed November 28, 2012).

American Physical Therapy Association. http://www.apta.org (accessed November 28, 2012).

American Psychiatric Association. http://www.psych.org (accessed November 28, 2012).

American Psychological Association. http://www.apa.org/ (accessed December 7, 2012).

American Society of Radiologic Technologists. http://www.asrt.org (accessed November 28, 2012).

American Speech-Language-Hearing Association. http://www.asha.org (accessed November 28, 2012).

American Yoga Association. http://www.americanyogaassociation.org (accessed November 28, 2012).

"Cause: Environment." *DoSomething.org.* http://www.dosomething.org/cause/environment (accessed November 12, 2012).

"Cause: Physical and Mental Health: Body Image." *DoSomething.org.* http://www.dosomething.org/cause/physical-and-mental-health (accessed November 12, 2012).

"Cause: Physical and Mental Health: Drug Abuse." *DoSomething.org.* http://www.dosomething.org/cause/physical-and-mental-health (accessed November 12, 2012).

Centers for Disease Control and Prevention. "Body, Facial & Dental Hygiene." http://www.cdc.gov/healthywater/hygiene/body/ (accessed October 24, 2012).

Centers for Disease Control and Prevention. "Handwashing: Clean Hands Save Lives." http://www.cdc.gov/handwashing (accessed October 24, 2012).

Centers for Disease Control and Prevention. "Lesbian, Gay, Bisexual and Transgender Health." http://www.cdc.gov/lgbthealth/youth.htm (accessed November 8, 2012).

Centers for Disease Control and Prevention. "Sexual Risk Behavior: HIV, STD, & Teen Pregnancy Prevention." http://www.cdc.gov/healthyyouth/sexualbehaviors/index.htm (accessed November 8, 2012).

Centers for Disease Control and Prevention. "Sexually Transmitted Diseases (STDs)." http://www.cdc.gov/std/default.htm (accessed November 8, 2012).

Centers for Disease Control and Prevention. "Teen Pregnancy." http://www.cdc.gov/TeenPregnancy/index.htm (accessed November 8, 2012).

"Child and Adolescent Mental Health." *National Institute of Mental Health (NIMH).* http://www.nimh.nih.gov/health/topics/child-and-adolescent-mental-health/index.shtml (accessed December 7, 2012).

Children's Environmental Health Network. http://www.cehn.org (accessed November 12, 2012).

ChooseMyPlate.gov. http://www.choosemyplate.gov (accessed October 29, 2012).

Earth Force. http://www.earthforce.org (accessed November 12, 2012).

"Eat Healthy." *LetsMove.gov.* http://www.letsmove.gov/eat-healthy (accessed October 29, 2012).

"Eating Disorders." *National Institute of Mental Health (NIMH).* http://www.nimh.nih.gov/health/topics/eating-disorders/index.shtml (accessed December 27, 2012).

Environmental Health Coalition. http://www.environmentalhealth.org (accessed November 12, 2012).

Families USA. http://www.familiesusa.org/ (accessed November 28, 2012).

Genetics Home Reference. http://ghr.nlm.nih.gov (accessed November 7, 2012).

GLAAD: Gay & Lesbian Advocates & Defenders. http://www.glaad.org/ (accessed November 8, 2012).

Healthfinder.gov. http://healthfinder.gov (accessed November 28, 2012).

Hey U.G.L.Y. (Unique Gifted Lovable You): Empowering Youth to Be a Part of the Solution to Bullying. http://www.heyugly.org/ (accessed December 7, 2012).

"How Regular Exercise Benefits Teens." *WebMD.com.* http://teens.webmd.com/benefits-of-exercise (accessed November 2, 2012).

Howard, Brian Clarke. "17 Easy Ways for Teens to Go Green." *TheDailyGreen.com.* http://www.thedailygreen.com/going-green/6334 (accessed November 12, 2012).

"Human Genome Project Information." *genomics.energy.gov.* http://www.ornl.gov/sci/techresources/Human_Genome/home.shtml (accessed November 7, 2012).

Let's Move. http://www.letsmove.gov/about (accessed November 2, 2012).

Mayo Clinic First Aid. http://www.mayoclinic.com/health/FirstAidIndex/FirstAidIndex (accessed November 16, 2012).

Mayo Clinic Food and Nutrition Center. "Nutrition and Healthy Eating." *MayoClinic.com.* http://www.mayoclinic.com/health/nutrition-and-healthy-eating/MY00431 (accessed October 29, 2012).

National Alliance on Mental Illness. http://www.nami.org (accessed December 11, 2012).

National Association for Self Esteem. http://www.self-esteem-nase.org (accessed December 7, 2012).

National Association of Emergency Medical Technicians. http://www.naemt.org (accessed November 28, 2012).

National Association of Social Workers. http://www.socialworkers.org (accessed November 28, 2012).

National Eating Disorders Association. http://www.nationaleatingdisorders.org/ (accessed December 27, 2012).

National Mental Health Association. http://www.nmha.org (accessed December 11, 2012).

The Nemours Foundation. "TeensHealth." *KidsHealth.org*. http://kidshealth.org/teen/ (accessed October 24, 2012).

The Nemours Foundation. "TeensHealth: Body Image and Self-Esteem." *KidsHealth.org* http://kidshealth.org/teen/food_fitness/wellbeing/body_image.html (accessed December 7, 2012).

The Nemours Foundation. "TeensHealth: Complementary and Alternative Medicine." *KidsHealth.org*. http://kidshealth.org/teen/your_body/medical_care/alternative_medicine.html (accessed November 28, 2012).

The Nemours Foundation. "TeensHealth: Drugs & Alcohol." *KidsHealth.org*. http://kidshealth.org/teen/drug_alcohol/ (accessed November 22, 2012).

The Nemours Foundation. "TeensHealth: Eating Disorders." *KidsHealth.org*. http://kidshealth.org/teen/food_fitness/problems/eat_disorder.html#cat20135 (accessed November 22, 2012).

The Nemours Foundation. "TeensHealth: Staying Safe." *KidsHealth.org*. http://kidshealth.org/teen/safety/ (accessed October 29, 2012).

The Nemours Foundation. "TeensHealth: Food and Fitness." *KidsHealth.org*. http://kidshealth.org/teen/food_fitness/ (accessed October 29, 2012).

The Nemours Foundation. "TeensHealth: Mind." *KidsHealth.org*. http://kidshealth.org/teen/your_mind (accessed December 7, 2012).

The Nemours Foundation. "TeensHealth: Prescription Drug Abuse." *KidsHealth.org*. http://kidshealth.org/teen/drug_alcohol/drugs/prescription_drug_abuse.html (accessed November 22, 2012).

The Nemours Foundation. "TeensHealth: Yoga." *KidsHealth.org*. http://kidshealth.org/teen/food_fitness/exercise/yoga.html (accessed November 28, 2012).

"NIDA for Teens: The Science Behind Drug Abuse" *U.S. National Institutes of Health: National Institute on Drug Abuse*. http://www.teens.drugabuse.gov (accessed December 27, 2012).

The Partnership at DrugFree.org. http://www.drugfree.org (accessed December 27, 2012).

Planned Parenthood. "Info for Teens." http://www.plannedparenthood.org/info-for-teens/ (accessed November 8, 2012).

"A Positive Image: Self-Esteem." *Palo Alto Medical Foundation*. http://www.pamf.org/teen/life/depression/selfesteem.html (accessed December 7, 2012).

President's Council on Fitness, Sports & Nutrition. "Be Active." *Fitness.gov*. http://www.fitness.gov (accessed November 2, 2012).

RAINN: Rape, Abuse & Incest National Network. http://centers.rainn.org/ (accessed November 9, 2012).

Reflexology Association of America. http://www.reflexology-usa.org (accessed November 28, 2012).

"The Science of Drug Abuse & Addiction." *U.S. National Institutes of Health: National Institute on Drug Abuse.* http://www.drugabuse.gov (accessed December 27, 2012).

"The Science of Drug Abuse & Addiction: Students and Young Adults." *U.S. National Institutes of Health: National Institute on Drug Abuse.* http://www.drugabuse.gov/students-young-adults (accessed December 27, 2012).

"Specific Genetic Disorders." *genome.gov.* http://www.genome.gov/1000120 (accessed November 7, 2012).

Substance Abuse and Mental Health Services Administration. http://www.samhsa.gov (accessed December 27, 2012).

"Teen Boy's Health." *WebMD.* http://teens.webmd.com/boys/default.htm (accessed November 16, 2012).

"The Teen Brain: Still Under Construction." *National Institute of Mental Health.* http://www.nimh.nih.gov/health/publications/the-teen-brain-still-under-construction/teens-and-the-brain-more-questions-for-research.shtml (accessed December 11, 2012).

"Teen Girl's Health." *WebMD.* http://teens.webmd.com/girls/default.htm (accessed November 16, 2012).

Teen Mental Health. http://www.teenmentalhealth.org/ (accessed December 7, 2012).

"Teen Mental Health." *Medline Plus.* http://www.nlm.nih.gov/medlineplus/teenmentalhealth.html (accessed December 7, 2012).

"Teen Survival Guide: Bullying." *girlshealth.gov.* http://www.girlshealth.gov/bullying/ (accessed December 7, 2012).

"Teen Survival Guide: Self-Esteem." *girlshealth.gov.* http://www.girlshealth.gov/teenguide/feelinggood/index.cfm (accessed December 7, 2012).

TeenGrowth.com. http://www.teengrowth.com/ (accessed November 7, 2012).

"Ten Self-Esteem Building Tips for Teens." *The Mental Health Association of South Central Kansas.* http://www.mhasck.org/news/article72.html (accessed December 7, 2012).

"Tween and Teen Health." *Mayo Clinic.* http://www.mayoclinic.com/health/tween-and-teen-health/MY00393 (accessed November 16, 2012).

University of Kansas Medical Center. "Genetics Education Center." http://www.kumc.edu/gec/ (accessed November 7, 2012).

U.S. Drug Enforcement Administration (DEA). http://www.justice.gov/dea/ (accessed November 19, 2012).

U.S. Environmental Protection Agency (EPA). "Site for Students". http://www.epa.gov/students (accessed November 12, 2012).

U.S. Environmental Protection Agency (EPA). "Your Environment: Your Choice." http://www.epa.gov/osw/education/teens/ (accessed November 12, 2012).

U.S. Food and Drug Administration (FDA). "Dietary Supplements Alerts." http://www.fda.gov/Food/DietarySupplements/Alerts/ (accessed August 15, 2012).

U.S. Food and Drug Administration (FDA). "Drugs." http://www.fda.gov/Drugs/default.htm (accessed August 15, 2012).

U.S. National Institute on Drug Abuse (NIDA). "NIDA for Teens." http://teens.drugabuse.gov/ (accessed November 21, 2012).

U.S. National Institute of Mental Health (NIMH). http://www.nimh.nih.gov (accessed December 7, 2012).

U.S. National Institutes of Health (NIH). "Homeopathy: An Introduction." *National Center for Complementary and Alternative Medicine (NCCAM).* http://nccam.nih.gov/health/homeopathy (accessed November 28, 2012).

U.S. National Institutes of Health (NIH). "Using Dietary Supplements Wisely." *National Center for Complementary and Alternative Medicine (NCCAM).* http://nccam.nih.gov/health/supplements/wiseuse.htm (accessed November 22, 2012).

U.S. National Institutes of Health (NIH). *National Center for Complementary and Alternative Medicine.* http://nih.gov (accessed November 28, 2012).

U.S. Substance Abuse and Mental Health Services Administration (SAMHSA). "Building Self-Esteem: A Self-Help Guide." https://store.samhsa.gov/shin/content//SMA-3715/SMA-3715.pdf (accessed December 7, 2012).

The Vegetarian Resource Group. http://www.vrg.org (accessed October 29, 2012).

"Your Body." *BAM! Body and Mind.* http://www.bam.gov/sub_yourbody/index.html (accessed October 24, 2012).

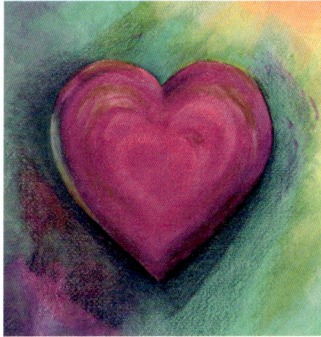

General Index

Page numbers in **boldface** indicate the main essay for a topic, and primary source page numbers are in ***boldface and italics***. An *italicized* page number indicates a photo, illustration, chart, or other graphic.

A

AA (Alcoholics Anonymous), *3:* 479
AAP (American Academy of Pediatrics), *2:* 252
Abdul, Paula, *3:* 570
Abortion, *1:* 172–174, 173 (ill.), 174 (ill.)
Abuse, *3:* 412, 420–421
ACA (Patient Protection and Affordable Care Act), *2:* 313, 316, 317, 317 (ill.)
Acetaminophen, *2:* 284, 298
Acid rain, *2:* 195–196
Acne, *1:* 85–86, 86 (ill.), 87 (ill.)
Acne medicines, *2:* 286
Acupuncture, *2:* 331 (ill.), 332, 385–388, 387 (ill.), 393, *3:* 557
Acupuncture model, *2:* 387
ADD (Attention-deficit disorder), *3:* 465
Addams, Jane, *2:* 362
Adderall (dextroamphetamine), *2:* 276
Addictions. *See also* **Behaviors, habits, addictions, and eating disorders**
    exercise, *1:* 74–75, *3:* 560–561, 573
    Internet, *3:* 559–560
    sugar, *3:* 555
    treatment, *3:* 554–558
ADHD (Attention-deficit / hyperactivity disorder), *1:* 141, *3:* 488–491, 490 (ill.), 494
Adler, Alfred, *3:* 457, 462
Adlerian psychology, *3:* 457, 459

Adolescence
    group therapy, *3:* 477 (ill.)
    growth and development during, *1:* 132, 132 (ill.), 134 (ill.), 134–135, 137 (ill.), 137–138
    self-esteem, *3:* 405, 408 (ill.), 415
Adoption, *1:* 123, 123 (ill.), 172, 174–175, *3:* 410
Adulthood, *1:* 132
Advanced practice nurses, *2:* 269, 359 (ill.), 359–361, *3:* 458 (ill.)
Aerobic dance, *1:* 56–57
Agoraphobia, *3:* 513–514
Agriculture, *2:* 192, 193–194, 194 (ill.)
AIDS/HIV, *1:* 166, 168, 175–176
Air pollution, indoor, *2:* 199–212, 201 (ill.), 204 (ill.), 206 (ill.), 209–212, 210 (ill.), 211 (ill.)
Air pollution, outdoor, *1:* 195–199, 196 (ill.)
Alba, Jessica, *1:* 52, *3:* 570
Alcohol and alcoholism
    alcohol abuse, *3:* 551–552
    drunk driving, *3:* 552, 552 (ill.)
    eating disorders and, *3:* 576
    effects of alcohol, *3:* 550–551, 551 (ill.)
    effects of alcohol abuse and addiction, *3:* 534, 552–553
    moderate consumption, *2:* 226–227
    peer pressure, *3:* 538–539
    sleep, *2:* 235
    water activities, *2:* 246
Alcoholics Anonymous (AA), *3:* 479
Alexander, Gabriel, *3:* 455

All Souls Cemetery (Chardon, OH), *3:* 421 (ill.)

Allergies, *2:* 202, 230–231, 395

Allergy medicines, *2:* 288 (ill.), 288–290, 297

Allopaths, *2:* 374

Alpha radiation, *2:* 189

Alternative medicine, *2:* 367–402. *See also*
  Mainstream medical system
    acupuncture, *2:* 331 (ill.), 332, 385–388,
      387 (ill.), 393
    Ayurvedic medicine, *2:* 397 (ill.), 397–398
    chiropractic, *2:* 331–332, 388–391, 390 (ill.)
    experimental, *2:* 332
    homeopathy, *2:* 369–376, 372 (ill.), 375 (ill.), 380
    mainstream medicine and, *2:* 331
    massage therapy, *2:* 391 (ill.), 391–394
    mental health therapy techniques, *3:* 467 (ill.),
      467–473, 472 (ill.)
    naturopathy, *2:* 332, 376–381, 377 (ill.)
    reflexology, *2:* 392, 394–397, 395 (ill.), 396 (ill.)
    traditional Chinese medicine, *2:* 380, 381–385,
      382 (ill.), 383 (ill.)
    yoga, *1:* 66–67, 74 (ill.), 159, *2:* 398–401,
      400 (ill.)

AMA (American Medical Association), *2:* 374, 379

American Academy of Child and Adolescent
  Psychiatry, *1:* 28 (ill.), *3:* 492

American Academy of Pediatrics (AAP), *2:* 252

American Association of Poison Control Centers
  (AAPCC), *2:* 209

American Institute of Homeopathy, *2:* 374

American Medical Association (AMA), *2:* 374, 379

American Psychiatric Association, *3:* 506, 516

Amphetamines, *3:* 544

Analgesics (pain relievers), *2:* 282–284, 283 (ill.)

Analytical psychology, *3:* 455–456

Anatomy
    female, *1:* 153–154
    male, *1:* 149–150

Anemia, *1:* 21, *2:* 237

Anesthesiology, *2:* 350

Animal-assisted therapy, *3:* 475 (ill.)

Anorexia nervosa, *1:* 31, *3:* 564–565, 566, 571 (ill.),
  571–572

Anorexic persons, *3:* 571 (ill.)

Antacids, *2:* 279–280

Anthony, Marc, *3:* 503

Anti-anxiety drugs and sleep aids, *3:* 540–541

Antibacterial agents, *2:* 285

Anti-Defamation League, *3:* 425

Antidiarrhea medicine, *2:* 281

Antihistamines medicine, *2:* 288–290

Antioxidants, *2:* 225–226, 253

Antiperspirants and deodorants, *1:* 83, 84 (ill.)

Antipsychotic drugs, *3:* 510

Anxiety disorders, *3:* 511–521, 514 (ill.), 517 (ill.),
  520 (ill.), 540–541

Apple, Fiona, *3:* 570

Arachnophobia therapy clinic, *3:* 514 (ill.)

Arkeen, Aaron West, *3:* 537

Arquette, David, *3:* 505

Art therapists, *2:* 335–336

Art therapy, *2:* 336 (ill.), *3:* 470

Asanas, *2:* 399

Asbestos, *2:* 206 (ill.), 206–207, 211

Asperger syndrome, *1:* 140, *3:* 498

Aspirin, *2:* 282–283, 297–298

Asthma
    acupuncture, *2:* 386
    air pollution, *2:* 202
    coffee, *2:* 283
    cold/flu medicines, *2:* 291
    environmental tobacco smoke, *2:* 200
    ephedra, *2:* 307
    food allergies, *2:* 230
    ginkgo, *2:* 384
    homeopathy, *2:* 376
    massage therapy, *2:* 391
    mobile medical apps, *2:* 329
    nitrogen dioxide exposure, *2:* 204
    reflexology, *2:* 395
    support groups, *2:* 329
    telemedicine, *2:* 329
    vitamins and minerals, *2:* 225
    yoga, *2:* 401

Athlete's foot, *1:* 91, 91 (ill.)

Attention-deficit disorder (ADD), *3:* 465

Attention-deficit / hyperactivity disorder (ADHD),
  1: 141, *3:* 488–491, 490 (ill.), 494

Auditory processing disorder, *1:* 141

Auricular acupuncture, *2:* 386, 395

Auscultation, *2:* 237
Autism spectrum disorder (ASD), *1:* 139–140, *3:* 498–501, 499 (ill.)
Ayurvedic medicine, *2:* 397 (ill.), 397–398

B

Bad breath, *1:* 97
Barbecued food, *2:* 226
BARCC (Boston Area Rape Crisis Center), *1:* 181 (ill.)
Barrymore, Drew, *3:* 537
Baseball, *1:* 69
Bateman, Justine, *3:* 570
Bath salts, *3:* 549
Bayer, *2:* 297
BDD (Body dysmorphic disorder), *3:* 521
Beans, *1:* 8 (ill.)
Beck, Aaron, *3:* 461, 462
Beckham, Victoria, *3:* 570
Beckinsale, Kate, *3:* 570
Bed-wetting, *3:* 502
Bedding care, *1:* 111
Behavior therapy, *3:* 462
Behavioral medicine, *3:* 465–466
Behaviors, habits, addictions, and eating disorders, *3:* 529–583
    addiction, *3:* 531, 534–535
    alcohol and alcoholism, *3:* 550–553, 551 (ill.), 552 (ill.), 576
    anti-anxiety drugs and sleep aids, *3:* 540–541
    body image, *3:* 575–576, 575 (ill.), 580–581
    caffeine, *3:* 554
    compulsive behaviors, *3:* 558–563, 559 (ill.), 561 (ill.)
    depressants, *3:* 539–543, 542 (ill.)
    eating disorders, *3:* 563–581, 565 (ill.), 571 (ill.), 575 (ill.)
    eating disorders and a positive body image, *3:* 580–581
    eating disorders and other destructive behaviors, *3:* 576
    eating disorders and sexuality, *3:* 576–577
    eating disorders causes, *3:* 567–571
    eating disorders consequences, *3:* 571 (ill.), 571–576
    eating disorders prevention, *3:* 579–580
    eating disorders treatment and recovery, *3:* 577–579
    habit defined, *3:* 531
    hallucinogens, *3:* 547–550
    inhalants, *3:* 550
    nicotine, *3:* 553 (ill.), 553–554
    positive body image, *3:* 580–581
    stimulants, *3:* 543–546, 545 (ill.)
    substance abuse, *3:* 535–539, 537 (ill.), 576
    treatment for addiction, *3:* 386, 554–558, 557 (ill.)
Belushi, John, *3:* 537
Bennett, Jay, *3:* 537
Beta radiation, *2:* 189
Bike riding, *1:* 57–58, *2:* 199, 202, 203 (ill.)
Bike safety, *1:* 58
Binet, Alfred, *3:* 449
Binge-eating disorder, *3:* 566–567, 572–573, 576
Bioenergetics, *3:* 469–470
Biofeedback, *3:* 465
Bipolar disorders, *3:* 507 (ill.), 507–508
Birth, stages of, *1:* 119
Birth control, *1:* 167 (ill.), 167–171, 169 (ill.), 170 (ill.)
Birth-control pill, *1:* 168–169, 167 (ill.), 169 (ill.)
Bisexuality, *1:* 164
Bisphenol A (BPA), *2:* 214–216
Bites and stings, *2:* 248–249, 260
Black plague, *2:* 202
Blood pressure check, *2:* 237
Blues and anxiety, *1:* 54–55
Blunt, Emily, *3:* 503
Boating, *2:* 246–247, 247 (ill.)
Body dysmorphic disorder (BDD), *3:* 521
Body hair, *1:* 93 (ill.), 93–95
Body image, *1:* 29–31, 30 (ill.), *3:* 575–576, 575 (ill.), 580–581
Body mass index (BMI), *1:* 28–29
Body/mind therapy, *3:* 469–470
Body odor, *1:* 83
Body shape, *1:* 27
Body type, *1:* 27
Bones, *1:* 51–52
Boot camp, *1:* 63

Borderline personality disorder (BPD), *3:* 525 (ill.), 526
Boston, Alex, *3:* 424 (ill.)
Boston Area Rape Crisis Center (BARCC), *1:* 181 (ill.)
Botanical medicine, *2:* 380
Bowden, Katrina, *1:* 52
Boxing, *1:* 63–64
BPA (Bisphenol A), *2:* 214–216
BPD (Borderline personality disorder), *3:* 525 (ill.), 526
Brand, Russell, *1:* 52
Bread, cereal, rice, and pasta group, *1:* 14–15
Breakfast, *1:* 41
Breast development, *1:* 155 (ill.), 156
Breath, bad, *1:* 97
Breathing, *1:* 52–53
Brendon, Nicholas, *3:* 503
Bubonic plague, *2:* 202
Bulimia nervosa, *1:* 31, *3:* 564, 565–566, 572, 576
Bullying, *3:* 422–424, 423 (ill.), 424 (ill.)
Burn and cut prevention/treatment, *2:* 240–241, 260
Butter *vs.* margarine, *2:* 227

C

Caffeine, *2:* 292, 300, *3:* 534, 554
Calcium, *1:* 19, *2:* 254
Calories, *1:* 9, 11–12
CAM (Complementary and alternative medicine). *See* **Alternative medicine**
Cancer
    cervical, *1:* 179
    skin, *2:* 237
Carbohydrates, *1:* 7–8
Carbon monoxide (CO), *2:* 197, 198, 203, 243
Cardiology, *2:* 350
Cardiopulmonary resuscitation (CPR), *2:* 257–258, 259
Cardiovascular fitness, *1:* 48–49
Caro, Isabella, *3:* 570
Carpenter, Karen, *3:* 570
Carrey, Jim, *1:* 141
Cavities, *1:* 97
CBT (Cognitive-behavioral therapy), *3:* 464

CDC (Centers for Disease Control and Prevention). *See* Centers for Disease Control and Prevention (CDC)
Celebrities as role models, *3:* 448–449
Celebrities' fitness, *1:* 52
Celiac disease and gluten intolerance, *1:* 39–40
Cells, *1:* 116–119
Center for Drug Evaluation and Research, *2:* 278
Center for Online Addiction, *3:* 559
Centers for Disease Control and Prevention (CDC)
    alcohol consumption, *2:* 227
    aspirin, *2:* 298
    blood lead levels, *2:* 207
    Down syndrome, *3:* 497, 497 (ill.)
    exercise, *1:* 45
    hand washing, *1:* 82
    obesity, *1:* 6
    physical activities and exercise, *1:* 45
    sugary drinks, *1:* 11
    violence, *3:* 421–422, 425
Centro de Salud (Phoenix, AZ), *2:* 316 (ill.)
Certified nurse-midwives (CNMs), *2:* 360
Cervarix, *1:* 179
Cervical cancer, *1:* 179
Cervical caps, *1:* 169
Character, *1:* 128–130
Childhood disintegrative disorder, *3:* 498
Childhood mental disorders, *3:* 487–503
    attention-deficit / hyperactivity disorder (ADHD), *3:* 488–491, 490 (ill.)
    autism, *3:* 498–501, 499 (ill.)
    autism spectrum disorder (ASD), *1:* 139–140, *3:* 498–501, 499 (ill.)
    bed-wetting, *3:* 502
    conduct disorders, *3:* 491–493, 492 (ill.)
    learning disorders, *1:* 140–141, *3:* 446, 494–495
    mental retardation, *1:* 139, *3:* 496–498, 497 (ill.)
    oppositional defiant disorder, *3:* 493–494
    stuttering, *3:* 502–503
    Tourette syndrome, *3:* 501
Children and exercise, *1:* 59
Children's Defense Fund, *2:* 243
Chimneys, stoves, heaters, and fireplaces, *2:* 202, 210–211
Chinese massage, *2:* 391 (ill.)
Chinese medicine, *2:* 380, 381–385, 382 (ill.), 383 (ill.)

Chiropractic, *2:* 331–332, 388–391, 390 (ill.)

Chlamydia, *1:* 176

Choking, *2:* 258 (ill.), 258–259

Cholesterol, *1:* 21

Cholesterol levels, *2:* 237

Choose MyPlate, *1:* 12–22, 13 (ill.)

CHPA (Consumer Healthcare Products Association), *2:* 278

Chromosomes, *1:* 117–118

Chronic medical conditions, *2:* 326–331, 327 (ill.), 329 (ill.)

Circumcised and uncircumcised penises, *1:* 108–110, 109 (ill.), 150–151, 152, 152 (ill.)

Clarkson, Kelly, *3:* 570

Classical conditioning, *3:* 446

Classroom presentations, *3:* 416 (ill.)

Clean Air Act, *2:* 187

Clinical nutrition, *2:* 380

Clitoris, *1:* 153

Clothing care, *1:* 110–111

Club drugs, *1:* 182

Clubs and drugs, *3:* 545

CNMs (Certified nurse-midwives), *2:* 360

Cocaine, *3:* 545–546

Cognitive-behavioral therapy (CBT), *3:* 464, 578

Cold medicines, *2:* 288, 288 (ill.), 290–291, 297

Collective unconscious, *3:* 455, 456

Collins, Francis, *1:* 120 (ill.)

Colognes, perfumes, and scented soaps and lotions, *1:* 83

Comaneci, Nadia, *3:* 570

Comfrey (*Symphytum officinale*), *2:* 307

Communication, *1:* 126–127

Complementary and alternative medicine (CAM). *See* **Alternative medicine**

Comprehensive Drug Abuse Prevention and Control Act, *2:* 275

Compulsive behaviors, *3:* 558–563, 559 (ill.), 561 (ill.)

Compulsive shopping, *3:* 562–563

Computerized tomography (CT), *2:* 358

Conception, *1:* 118, 154

Conditioner and shampoo, *1:* 91–92

Conditioning, *3:* 446–447, 447 (ill.)

Condoms, *1:* 167 (ill.), 167–168, 169 (ill.), 179

Conduct disorders, *3:* 491–493, 493 (ill.)

Congress, *2:* 187, 275, *3:* 549

Consciousness, *3:* 456

Consumer Healthcare Products Association (CHPA), *2:* 278

Contraceptives
cervical cap, *1:* 169
condoms, *1:* 167 (ill.), 167–168, 169 (ill.), 179
diaphragms, *1:* 169
emergency, *1:* 171
implants, *1:* 170
injectable, *1:* 170
intrauterine devices (IUDs), *1:* 167 (ill.), 169–170, 170 (ill.)
oral, *1:* 167 (ill.), 168–169, 169 (ill.)
patches, *1:* 167 (ill.), 170–171

Convergent thinkers, *3:* 450–451

Copper in diet, *2:* 254

CORA Services (Philadelphia, PA), *3:* 553 (ill.)

Cortisone/Hydrocortisone, *2:* 285–286

Cough medicines, *2:* 288, 288 (ill.), 290–291

Couric, Katie, *3:* 570

CPR (cardiopulmonary resuscitation), *2:* 257–258, 259

Crabs (pubic lice), *1:* 180

Cramps (dysmenorrhea), *1:* 159

Creative art therapies, *3:* 470–472, 472 (ill.)

Creativity, *3:* 450–452, 451 (ill.)

Cruise, Suri, *1:* 52

Crushes, *1:* 159–160

CT (computerized tomography), *2:* 358

Culture and language, *1:* 125–127, 145

Culture and mental illness, *3:* 485

Cut and burn prevention/treatment, *2:* 240–241, 260

Cuticles, *1:* 102, 102 (ill.)

Cutting, *3:* 561 (ill.), 561–562

Cyberbullying, *3:* 424, 424 (ill.)

D

Dairy product group, *1:* 17–18, 38, 38 (ill.), *2:* 256

Dance, *1:* 56–57, 58, 59 (ill.)

Dance and movement therapy, *3:* 471

Dandruff, *1:* 92–93

Danes, Claire, *3:* 499 (ill.)

Date rape, *1:* 182

Dating, *1:* 160

DEA (Drug Enforcement Administration), *3:* 549

Death, *3:* 478

Dechanel, Zooey, *1:* 141

Decongestant eye drops, *2:* 299

Decongestants, *2:* 288, 288 (ill.), 290, 298–299

Delusions, *3:* 508, 509

Dental and oral care, *1:* 95–98, 96 (ill.), 98 (ill.), *2:* 236, 236 (ill.)

Dentists, *1:* 95, 97–98, 98 (ill.), *2:* 336–338, 337 (ill.)

Deodorants and antiperspirants, *1:* 83, 84 (ill.)

Department of Agriculture (USDA), *1:* 6, 11, 16

Department of Defense (DOD), *2:* 192

Department of Education, *3:* 425

Department of Energy (DOE), *2:* 192

Department of Health and Human Services (HHS), *1:* 11, *2:* 192, 215, 275

Department of Transportation (DOT), *2:* 192

Dependence, *3:* 534–535

Dependent personality disorder, *3:* 525

Depilatories, *1:* 94

Depo-Provera, *1:* 170

Depressants, *3:* 539–543, 542 (ill.)

Depression, *3:* 502–507, 504 (ill.), 505, 574

Dermatologists and dermatology, *2:* 286, 350

DES (Diethylstilbestrol), *2:* 215

Desai, Nikita, *3:* 517 (ill.)

Designer drugs, *3:* 548–550

Development. *See* **Personal growth and development**

Developmental disorders, *1:* 139–141

Dextroamphetamine (Adderall), *2:* 276

Dey, Susan, *3:* 570

Diabetes, *2:* 327 (ill.)

Diagnostic and Statistical Manual of Mental Disorders (DSM–IV), *3:* 488–489, 498

Diana, Princess of Wales, *3:* 570

Diaphragms, *1:* 169

Diet, healthy, *2:* 224–229, *3:* 480

Diet pills, *1:* 33

Dietary Guidelines for Americans, *1:* 6, 11, *2:* 225

Dietary supplements and preventive medicine, *2:* 251–255

Dietary supplements and herbal remedies, *2:* 301–303, 302 (ill.), 303 (ill.), 306–308, 383–385

Diethylstilbestrol (DES), *2:* 215

Dieting, *1:* 31–34, *3:* 581

Dietitians, *2:* 338–339

Digestion drugs, *2:* 279–281

Dillingham, Kate, *3:* 472 (ill.)

Diphtheria-Tetanus-Pertussis (DTaP, DTP) vaccines, *2:* 238

Diseased human lung, *3:* 557 (ill.)

Disorder of written expression, *3:* 495

Dissociative disorders, *3:* 522–524, 524 (ill.)

Divergent thinkers, *3:* 450–451

Divorce and separation, *3:* 411

DNA, *1:* 117

Doctors of osteopathy (DOs), *2:* 269

DOD (Department of Defense), *2:* 192

DOE (Department of Energy), *2:* 192

Dog training, *3:* 447, 447 (ill.)

Doherty Middle School (Andover, MA), *1:* 34 (ill.)

DOs (Doctors of osteopathy), *2:* 269

DOT (Department of Transportation), *2:* 192

Douches and feminine hygiene sprays, *1:* 106–107

Down syndrome, *1:* 122, *3:* 497, 497 (ill.)

Dream analysis, *3:* 454

Drug abuse. *See* Substance abuse

Drug Enforcement Administration (DEA), *3:* 549

Drug therapy, *3:* 466–467

Drug use and injury, *2:* 246

Drugs. *See* **Medications;** *specific drugs*

Drunk driving, *3:* 552, 552 (ill.)

DSM-IV (Diagnostic and Statistical Manual of Mental Disorders), *3:* 488–489, 498

DTaP and DTP (Diphtheria-Tetanus-Pertussis) vaccines, *2:* 238

Duff, Haylie, *1:* 52

Duff, Hilary, *1:* 52, 141

Dyscalculia, *1:* 141, *3:* 495

Dysgraphia, *1:* 140

Dyslexia, *1:* 140, *3:* 495

Dysmenorrhea (cramps), *1:* 159

Dyspraxia, *1:* 141

E

Ear care, *1:* 98–101

Ear piercings, *1:* 99

Eating disorders, *3:* 563–581. *See also* **Behaviors, habits, addictions, and eating disorders**
    anorexia nervosa, *1:* 31, *3:* 564–565, 566, 571 (ill.), 571–572
    body image, *3:* 575–576, 575 (ill.), 580–581
    bulimia nervosa, *1:* 31, *3:* 564, 565–566, 572, 576
    causes, *3:* 567–571
    consequences of, *3:* 571 (ill.), 571–576
    males, *3:* 567
    overview, *1:* 31, *3:* 563–564
    persons with, *3:* 571 (ill.), 575 (ill.)
    positive body image, *3:* 580–581
    prevention, *3:* 579–580
    sexuality and, *3:* 576–577
    substance abuse, *3:* 576
    treatment and recovery, *3:* 577–579
Ecstasy (MDMA), *3:* 548
Eczema, *1:* 88
Ego, *3:* 454
Einstein, Albert, *3:* 495
Electricity safety, *2:* 245–246
Electrolysis, *1:* 94
Ellis, Albert, *3:* 464
Emergencies, medical, *2:* 324–326, 325 (ill.), 330
Emergency contraceptive pills, *1:* 171
Emergency medical technicians (EMTs), *2:* 269, 339–341, 340 (ill.)
Emergency rooms, *2:* 325 (ill.)
Emotional intelligence, *1:* 138–139
Emotional intimacy, *1:* 162 (ill.), 162–163
Emotions, *1:* 129
Empathy, *1:* 138, 139
EMTs (Emergency medical technicians), *2:* 269, 339–341, 340 (ill.)
Endocrine disrupters, *2:* 212–217, 214 (ill.)
Endorphins, *1:* 54
Energy and physical activity, *1:* 53
Entwistle, John, *3:* 537
Environment and development, *1:* 122–127, 123 (ill.), 124 (ill.), 125 (ill.), 126 (ill.)
Environmental estrogens, *2:* 213–214
Environmental health, *2:* 185–218
    endocrine disrupters, *2:* 212–217, 214 (ill.)
    indoor air pollution, *2:* 199–212, 201 (ill.), 204 (ill.), 205 (ill.), 206 (ill.), 211 (ill.)

    outdoor air pollution, *2:* 195–199, 196 (ill.), 198 (ill.)
    pesticides, *2:* 192–195, 194 (ill.), 208–209, 212
    radiation, *2:* 189–192, 190 (ill.)
Environmental medicine, *2:* 380
Environmental Protection Agency (EPA)
    pesticides, *2:* 195
    pollution, *2:* 187, 198, 199, 204, 206, 210
    radiation, *2:* 191, 192
Environmental tobacco smoke (ETS), *2:* 200–202, 210, 210 (ill.), 228
Environmental Working Group (EWG), *2:* 187
EPA (Environmental Protection Agency). *See* Environmental Protection Agency (EPA)
Ephedra (*Ephedra sinica*), *2:* 307–308
Epstein, Howie, *3:* 537
Equine (horse) therapy, *3:* 475 (ill.)
Erections, *1:* 151
Erikson, Erik, *1:* 131, 132 (ill.), *3:* 440–441
Estrogen, *1:* 154–155
ETS (Environmental tobacco smoke), *2:* 200–202, 210, 210 (ill.), 227
Everglades, *2:* 215
EWG (Environmental Working Group), *2:* 187
Exercise
    evolution of, *1:* 50
    and health, *2:* 231–232
    and memory, *3:* 443
    and mental health, *3:* 480
    types of, *1:* 49, 49 (ill.)
Exercise addiction, *1:* 74, *3:* 560–561
Existential therapy, *3:* 459
Experimental treatments, *2:* 332
Extreme sports, *1:* 67
Eye drops, *2:* 299
Eye protection, *2:* 250
Eyre, Scott, *1:* 141

F

Facebook, *3:* 424 (ill.), 425
Facial hair, *1:* 93, 93 (ill.)
Factitious disorders, *3:* 522
Fad diets, *1:* 32

Fall prevention, *2:* 240
Family
    death in the, *3:* 478
    drug abuse, *3:* 538–539
    eating disorders and, *3:* 569
    homosexuality, *1:* 163
    military deployment in the, *3:* 411, 472 (ill.)
    personal growth and development, *1:* 123 (ill.),
        123–124, 124 (ill.), 125 (ill.), 126 (ill.)
    self-concept/self-esteem and, *3:* 407, 408,
        409–412, 410 (ill.), 420
    therapy, *3:* 474–476, 475 (ill.), 578
Fanning, Dakota, *1:* 52
Farley, Chris, *3:* 537
Fat in diet, *1:* 6–7, 20–22, *2:* 226
Fears. *See* Phobias
Federal Insecticide, Fungicide, and Rodenticide Act
    (FIFRA), *2:* 195
Federal Trade Commission (FTC), *2:* 279
Fee-for-service health care, *2:* 318
Female anatomy, *1:* 153–154
Feminine hygiene products, *1:* 106–107, 107 (ill.)
Fetus, development of, *1:* 118–119, *2:* 214–216
Fiber in diet, *2:* 224–225
Fingernails, ringworm, *1:* 102–103
Firearm violence, *2:* 241–243, 242 (ill.)
Firearm safety, *2:* 242, 242 (ill.)
Fireplaces, stoves, heaters, and chimneys, *2:* 202,
    210–211
First aid, *2:* 256–261, 257 (ill.), 258 (ill.), 259 (ill.)
First aid kits, *2:* 257 (ill.), 259 (ill.), 259–260, 291
Fitness, *See* Physical Fitness and Exercise *and* Sports
Fitzgerald, William, *2:* 395
Flexibility, *1:* 53
Flockheart, Calista, *3:* 570
Flossing, *1:* 96 (ill.), 96–97
Flu medicine, *2:* 288, 290–291
Flu shots, *2:* 239
Fonda, Jane, *3:* 570
Food. *See also* **Nutrition**
    barbecued, *2:* 226
    and feelings, *1:* 30
    food groups, *1:* 11
    fried, *1:* 26 (ill.), *2:* 226
    processed, *2:* 226
    safety, *2:* 230
    smoked, *2:* 226
    takeout, *1:* 26 (ill.)
Food allergies and intolerance, *1:* 37–40, 38 (ill.),
    2: 230–231
Food and Drug Administration (FDA)
    acetaminophen, *2:* 298
    BPA, *2:* 215
    dietary supplements, *2:* 301–302, 307,
        307–308
    drug patents, *2:* 271
    emergency contraception, *1:* 171
    homeopathic remedies regulation, *2:* 376
    OTC medications, *2:* 296–297, 304
    over-the-counter drugs, *2:* 278
    radiation, *2:* 191
    sunscreens, *1:* 87, 88
    tamper-evident packaging, *2:* 304
Food groups, *1:* 11
Food safety, *2:* 230
Foot protection, *2:* 249
Football, *1:* 71 (ill.)
Foster children, *3:* 410
Francis of Assisi, Saint, *1:* 83
Free association, *3:* 454
French, Morton, *3:* 455
Freud, Sigmund, *3:* 453, 453 (ill.), 455
Fried food, *1:* 26 (ill.), *2:* 226
Friends
    making and keeping, *3:* 419
    physical activities with, *1:* 69–70
    self-esteem and, *3:* 417, 418 (ill.), 420–421
Fruits and vegetables, *1:* 25 (ill.)
    in diet, *1:* 15–17, 16 (ill.), 17 (ill.), *2:* 225,
        226 (ill.)
    fruit group, *1:* 16, 16 (ill.), 17, 17 (ill.)
    snacks, *1:* 5 (ill.), 17 (ill.)
    vegetable group, *1:* 15, 16 (ill.)

G

GAD (Generalized anxiety disorder), *3:* 512
Gambling, *3:* 559
Gamma radiation, *2:* 190–191

Gardasil, *1:* 179–180
Gardnerella, *1:* 104
Garland, Judy, *3:* 537
Garrison, Zina, *3:* 570
Gastroenterology, *2:* 350
Gein, Gidget, *3:* 537
Gender, *1:* 145
Gene therapy, *1:* 122
Generalized anxiety disorder (GAD), *3:* 512
Generic drugs, *2:* 269–271
Genes, *1:* 117–118
Genetic disorders, *1:* 122, *3:* 496
Genetic testing, *1:* 121
Genetic variation, *1:* 120
Genetics, *1:* 27–28, 116–122, 117 (ill.)
Genital care
    females, *1:* 103–107, 107 (ill.)
    males, *1:* 108–110, 109 (ill.)
Genital warts, *1:* 179
Genome, human, *1:* 119–120
Genomic medicine, *1:* 121
Gestalt therapy, *3:* 460–461
GHB, *1:* 182
Ginseng (panax ginseng), *2:* 308
Girls, Inc., *1:* 148 (ill.)
Glasser, William, *3:* 466
Gluten intolerance and celiac disease, *1:* 39–40
Gold, Tracey, *3:* 570
Gonorrhea, *1:* 177
Goudreault, Francois, *3:* 503
Graham, Sylvester, *2:* 371
Grain group, *1:* 14–15
Grandin, Temple, *3:* 499, 499 (ill.)
Gray, Paul, *3:* 537
Great Lakes area, *2:* 215
Great Lakes Naval Station, *3:* 472 (ill.)
Greene, Ashley, *1:* 52
Gregory IX (pope), *1:* 83
Groin ringworm. *See* Jock itch
Group therapy, *3:* 476–479, 477 (ill.), 578–579
Growing Together workshop, *1:* 148 (ill.)
Growth. *See* **Personal growth and development**
Guenther, Heidi, *3:* 570
Gull, William, *3:* 564
Gum disease, *1:* 97

Guns and gun violence, *2:* 241–243, *3:* 421–422,
    421 (ill.)
Gymnastics, *1:* 53 (ill.), 58–59
Gynecology, *2:* 350

H

H_2-antagonists, *2:* 280–281
Habits. *See* **Behaviors, habits, addictions, and
    eating disorders**
Haemophilus influenzae type b (Hib), *2:* 238
Hahnemann, Samuel, *2:* 371–373
Haim, Corey, *3:* 537
Hair care, *1:* 88–95, 92 (ill.)
Hair removal, 1: 93–95
Hale, Lucy, *3:* 570
Halitosis. *See* Bad breath
Halliwell, Geri, *3:* 570
Hallucinations, *3:* 508, 509, 510
Hallucinogens, *3:* 547–550
Hamm, Jon, *3:* 505
Hand washing, *1:* 81–82, 82 (ill.), *2:* 236
Head injuries, *1:* 70–71, 71 (ill.)
Head lice, *1:* 92, 92 (ill.)
Health care system. *See* **Mainstream medical
    system**
Health maintenance organizations (HMOs),
    2: 319–321, 324, 330
Health Resources and Services Administration,
    3: 425
Health service administrators, *2:* 341–343
Hearing, *1:* 100–101
Hearing and vision tests, *2:* 239
Heat exhaustion, *2:* 261
Heaters, fireplaces, stoves, and chimneys, *2:* 202,
    210–211
Heidegger, Martin, *3:* 459
Heimlich maneuver, *2:* 258 (ill.), 258–259
Helmets and sports, *1:* 58, 60, 69, 70–71, 71 (ill.),
    2: 249
Hemingway, Margaux, *3:* 570
Hemorrhoid medicine, *2:* 287–288
Hendrix, Jimi, *3:* 537
Henrich, Christy, *3:* 570

Hepatitis A (HepA), *2:* 238

Hepatitis B (HepB), *2:* 238

Herbal remedies and dietary supplements,
2: 251–255, 301–303, 302 (ill.), 303 (ill.),
306–308, 383–385

Hering, Constantine, *2:* 373, 375–376

Herman, Jarred, *3:* 475 (ill.)

Herman family, *3:* 475 (ill.)

Heroic medicine, *2:* 373

Herpes, *1:* 178

HHS (Department of Health and Human Services),
1: 11, *2:* 192, 215, 275

High blood pressure, *2:* 237

High school staff, *3:* 557 (ill.)

Hiking, *1:* 59–60, *2:* 232 (ill.)

Hippocrates, *2:* 374

HIV/AIDS, *1:* 166, 168, 175–176

HMOs (Health maintenance organizations),
2: 319–321, 324, 330

Hobbies and stress, *2:* 234

Holmes, Katie, *1:* 52

Homeopathy, *2:* 369–376, 372 (ill.), 375 (ill.),
380

Homophobia, *1:* 164

Homosexuality, *1:* 163

Hooker, John Lee, *3:* 503

Hooking up, *1:* 161–162

Hoon, Shannon, *3:* 537

Hormonal implants, *1:* 170, 170 (ill.)

Hormones, *1:* 149, 154–155, 167 (ill.), *2:* 212–217,
214 (ill.)

Horse (equine) therapy, *3:* 475 (ill.)

Household injuries, *2:* 239–241

Household products, *2:* 204–205, 205 (ill.), 211,
211 (ill.)

Houston, Whitney, *3:* 537

HPV (Human papilloma virus), *1:* 178–180,
179 (ill.) *2:* 237, 238

Hudgens, Vanessa, *1:* 52

Hull House (Chicago, IL), *2:* 362

Human genome, *1:* 119–120

Human papilloma virus (HPV), *1:* 178–180,
179 (ill.) *2:* 237, 238

Humanistic and existential therapies, *3:* 455–459

Hydration, *1:* 10, 10 (ill.), *2:* 229 (ill.)

Hydrocortisone/Cortisone, *2:* 285–286

Hygiene. *See* **Personal care and hygiene**

Hymen, *1:* 153, 154

Hypnotherapy, *3:* 473

Hypothermia, *2:* 261

I

Ibuprofen, *2:* 284

ICD-10 (International Statistical Classification of
Diseases, Injuries, and Causes of Death), *3:* 488

Ice skating, *1:* 60

Id, *3:* 453

Illness in family, *3:* 411

Illness prevention
diet, *2:* 224–227, 228–229
exercise, *2:* 231–232, 232 (ill.)
food allergies and intolerance, *2:* 230–231
food safety, *2:* 230
hygiene practices, *2:* 236
physical examination and check-ups,
2: 236–239, 238 (ill.)
sleep, *2:* 234–236, 235 (ill.)
smoking, *2:* 227–228
stress management, *2:* 232–234
water consumption, *2:* 228, 229 (ill.)

Immunizations, *2:* 236, 238, 238 (ill.), 239

Improving Your Memory (Stern), *3:* 443

In-line skating, *1:* 60, 69 (ill.)

Inactivated poliovirus vaccine (IPV), *2:* 238

Independent eaters, *1:* 35

Indigestion, *2:* 255–256

Individual therapy, *3:* 473–474

Individuality, *3:* 440–442

Indoor air pollution, *2:* 199–212, 201 (ill.),
204 (ill.), 206 (ill.), 209–212

Infancy, *1:* 131, 132, 135, *3:* 441

Influenza vaccines (TIV), *2:* 238

Ingham, Eunice, *2:* 395

Ingrown toenails, *1:* 101

Inhalants, *3:* 550

Injury prevention

electricity safety, *2:* 245–246

gun violence, *2:* 241–243, 242 (ill.)

household injuries, *2:* 239–241

outdoor injuries, *2:* 246–249, 247 (ill.), 250 (ill.)

poisoning, *2:* 243 (ill.), 243–245

sports injuries, *1:* 68–74

Insect bites and stings, *2:* 248–249, 260

Insight therapy

humanistic and existential therapies, *3:* 455–457, 459

psychoanalysis, *3:* 453–455

psychotherapy, *3:* 452

Insomnia, *2:* 294

Intellectual development, *1:* 135–138

Intelligence, *3:* 438, 439 (ill.), 449–450

Intelligence quotient (IQ), *3:* 449–450, 496

International Statistical Classification of Diseases, Injuries, and Causes of Death (ICD–10), *3:* 488

Internet

eating disorders, *3:* 577

Facebook, *3:* 424 (ill.), 425

Twitter, *3:* 425

Internet addiction, *3:* 559 (ill.), 559–560

Intervention, *3:* 556

Intimacy, *1:* 162 (ill.), 162–163

Intrauterine devices (IUDs), *1:* 167 (ill.), 169–170, 170 (ill.)

Ionizing radiation, *2:* 189

IPV (Inactivated poliovirus vaccine), *2:* 238

IQ (Intelligence quotient), *3:* 449–450, 496

Iron in diet, *1:* 9, *2:* 254

Isabella of Spain, *1:* 83

IUDs (Intrauterine devices), *1:* 167 (ill.), 169–170, 170 (ill.)

J

Jackman, Hugh, *1:* 52

Jackson, Michael, *3:* 537

James River (Richmond, VA), *2:* 214 (ill.)

Jaspers, Karl, *3:* 459

Jock itch, *1:* 108

John, Elton, *3:* 570

Johns, Daniel, *3:* 570

Johnson, Kathy, *3:* 570

Joint health, *2:* 302

Jonas, Joe, *1:* 52

Jonas, Nick, *2:* 327 (ill.)

Jones, James Earl, *3:* 503

Joplin, Janis, *3:* 537

Judd, Ashley, *3:* 505

Judd, Winona, *3:* 570

Jung, Carl Gustav, *3:* 455–456, 457

Junk food, *1:* 22–23

Justice, Victoria, *1:* 52

K

Kardashian, Kim, *1:* 52

Kardashian, Kourtney, *1:* 52

Kava *(Piper methysticum)*, *2:* 308

Ketamine, *1:* 182, *3:* 548–549

Kidman, Nicole, *3:* 503

Kierkegaard, Soren, *3:* 459

King, B. B., *3:* 503

Kirkland, Gelsey, *3:* 570

Kissing, *1:* 160

Kleptomania, *3:* 562

Kneipp, Sebastian, *2:* 379

Knightley, Keira, *3:* 495

Knowles, Solange, *1:* 141

Koch, Robert, *1:* 83

Korzun, Adam, *2:* 226 (ill.)

Kournikova, Anna, *1:* 52

Kunis, Mila, *1:* 52

L

LaBeouf, Shia, *1:* 52

Lactose intolerance, *1:* 38, 38 (ill.), *2:* 231, 256

Lady Gaga, *3:* 570

Language and culture, *1:* 125

Lasegue, Charles, *3:* 564

Laser treatments for hair removal, *1:* 95

Lavigne, Avril, *1:* 141

Lawless, Lucy, *3:* 570

Laxatives, *2:* 281–282, 299–300

Lead, *2:* 197–198, 198 (ill.), 199, 207–208, 208 (ill.), 211, 244, 244 (ill.)

Learning, *3:* 444–449, 447 (ill.), 448 (ill.)

Learning disorders, *1:* 140–141, *3:* 446, 494–495

Leary, Timothy, *3:* 547

Ledger, Heath, *3:* 537

Legumes, *1:* 8 (ill.)

Lentils, *1:* 8 (ill.)

Leonardo da Vinci, *3:* 495

Levine, Adam, *1:* 141

Levonorgestrel tablets, *1:* 171

Lice, *1:* 92, 92 (ill.), 180

Lillard, Harvey, *2:* 389

London, Stacy, *3:* 570

Los Angeles Fire Department EMTs, *2:* 340 (ill.)

Lotions and soaps, *1:* 83

Lovato, Demi, *1:* 52, *3:* 505, 507 (ill.), 570

Lowen, Alexander, *3:* 469

LSD (Lysergic acid diethylamide), *3:* 547

Ludes, *3:* 541

Lust, Benedict, *2:* 379

Lutz, Keilan, *1:* 52

Lysergic acid diethylamide (LSD), *3:* 547

M

Magnesium in diet, *2:* 254

Magnetic resonance imaging (MRI), *2:* 355, 356, 357 (ill.)

Main, Amber, *3:* 510 (ill.)

Mainstream medical system, *2:* 311–365. See also **Alternative medicine**

    advanced practice nurses, *2:* 269, 359 (ill.), 359–361, *3:* 458 (ill.)

    art therapists, *2:* 335–336

    chronic conditions, *2:* 326–331, 327 (ill.), 329 (ill.)

    computerized tomography (CT), *2:* 358

    dentists, *2:* 336–338, 337

    dermatologists, *2:* 286

    dietitians, *2:* 338–339

    doctors of osteopathy (DOs), *2:* 269

    emergencies, *2:* 324–326, 330

    emergency medical technicians, *2:* 269, 339–341, 340 (ill.)

    health care careers, *2:* 335

    health service administrators, *2:* 341–343

    health system defined, *2:* 316–317

    licensed health care professionals, *2:* 269–271, 271 (ill.)

    managed care *vs.* fee-for-service, *2:* 318–322, 321 (ill.)

    Medicaid, *2:* 324

    medical assistants, *2:* 316 (ill.)

    Medicare, *2:* 322–323

    mental health counselors, *2:* 343–344

    nuclear medicine technologists, *2:* 358

    occupational therapists, *2:* 344–345

    optometrists, *2:* 269, 345–346, 346 (ill.)

    orthodontists, *2:* 337 (ill.)

    patient advocates, *2:* 342

    pharmacists, *2:* 269, 271 (ill.), 347 (ill.), 347–348

    physical therapists, *2:* 348–349, 349 (ill.)

    physician assistants (PAs), *2:* 269, 359–361

    physicians, *2:* 269, 320, 321 (ill.), 349–352, 351 (ill.)

    psychologists, *2:* 269, 352–355

    radiological technologists, *2:* 355–358, 357 (ill.)

    registered nurses, *2:* 358–361, 359 (ill.)

    social workers, *2:* 269, 361–362

    speech language pathologists, *2:* 362–363

    substance abuse and mental health problems, *2:* 333–334

    substance abuse counselors, *2:* 344

Major depression, *3:* 503–507, 504 (ill.)

Makeup, *1:* 88, 90 (ill.)

Male anatomy, *1:* 149–150

The Man Who Mistook His Wife for a Hat (Sacks), *3:* 500

Managed health care, *2:* 318–322, 321 (ill.)

Mandel, Howie, *1:* 141

Manias, *3:* 562

Manicures and pedicures, *1:* 101

Mantras, *3:* 558

Margarine *vs.* butter, *2:* 227

Marijuana, *3:* 541–543, 542 (ill.)

Marriage and family therapy, *3:* 474–476, 475 (ill.), 578

Marshall, Brandon, *3:* 525 (ill.)

Martial arts, *1:* 60–61, 61 (ill.)

Mary Mitchell Family & Youth Center, *1:* 61 (ill.)

Massage therapy, *2:* 391 (ill.), 391–394

Masturbation, *1:* 166

Mathematical learning disorder, *1:* 141, *3:* 495

MCAT (Medical College Admission Test), *2:* 352

McConaughey, Matthew, *1:* 52

MCV4 (Meningococcal conjugate vaccines, quadrivalent), *2:* 238

MDMA (Ecstasy), *3:* 548

Meal supplements, *2:* 302

Measles-Mumps-Rubella (MMR), *2:* 238

Media, impact of, *3:* 409, 580

Medicaid, *2:* 324

Medical College Admission Test (MCAT), *2:* 352

Medical marijuana, *3:* 541–543, 542 (ill.)

Medical students, *2:* 351 (ill.)

Medical system. *See* **Mainstream medical system**

Medicare, *2:* 322–323

Medications, *2:* 263–310
  dietary supplements and herbal remedies, *2:* 301–303, 302 (ill.), 303 (ill.), 306–308
  drug delivery routes, *2:* 268
  licensed health care professionals, *2:* 269–271, 271 (ill.)
  over-the-counter drugs, *2:* 277, 278–279, 303–305, 305 (ill.), 308 (ill.), *3:* 539
  over-the-counter drugs, common types, *2:* 279–291, 283 (ill.), 285 (ill.), 288 (ill.)
  over-the-counter drugs, controversial or potentially dangerous, *2:* 292–301
  overdoses and missed doses, *2:* 272–274
  prescription, *2:* 267–274, 271 (ill.), 273 (ill.), 296–297, 308 (ill.), 329–330, *3:* 539
  prescription drug abuse, *2:* 274–278, 277 (ill.)
  safety, *2:* 244–245, 303–309, 305 (ill.), 308 (ill.)
  types of, *2:* 265–266

Medicine, behavioral, *3:* 465

Medicine cabinet safety, *2:* 244–245

Medigap, *2:* 323

Meditation, *2:* 400 (ill.), *3:* 467, 468–469, 557–558

Meditative asanas, *2:* 398–399

Memory, *3:* 442–444

Meningococcal conjugate vaccines, quadrivalent (MCV4), *2:* 238

Menstruation, *1:* 105–106, 107 (ill.), 156–159, 157 (ill.), 172

Mental health, *3:* 433–481
  becoming an individual, *3:* 440–442
  choosing a therapist, *3:* 458, 458 (ill.)
  cognitive and behavior therapies, *3:* 461–466, 463 (ill.)
  creativity, *3:* 450–452, 451 (ill.)
  insight therapy, *3:* 452–461
  intelligence, *3:* 449–450
  learning, *3:* 444–449, 448 (ill.)
  memory, *3:* 442–444
  nature *vs.* nurture, *3:* 436–440
  nontraditional mental health therapy techniques, *3:* 467 (ill.), 467–473, 472 (ill.)
  pharmacotherapy, *3:* 466–467
  psychotherapy, *3:* 452, 452 (ill.)
  self-help, *3:* 480
  therapies, *3:* 452
  therapy formats, *3:* 473–479, 475 (ill.), 477 (ill.)

Mental health counselors, *2:* 343–344

Mental health treatment, *2:* 333–334

Mental illness, *3:* 483–527
  anxiety disorders, *3:* 511–521, 514 (ill.), 517 (ill.), 520 (ill.), 540–541
  childhood disorders, *3:* 487–503, 490 (ill.)
  dissociative disorders, *3:* 522–524, 524 (ill.)
  mood disorders, *3:* 503–508, 504 (ill.), 507 (ill.)
  personality disorders, *3:* 524–526, 525 (ill.)
  psychotic disorders, *3:* 508–511, 510 (ill.)
  somatoform disorders, *3:* 521–522

Mental retardation, *1:* 139, *3:* 496–498, 497 (ill.)

Mescaline, *3:* 548

Meth ingredients (Union, MO), *3:* 545 (ill.)

Methadone maintenance, *3:* 556

Methamphetamines, *3:* 544–545, 545 (ill.)

Methylphenidate (Ritalin), *2:* 276

Midwives, *2:* 360

Migraine headaches, *2:* 229

Migrant workers, *2:* 351 (ill.)

Military deployment, *3:* 411, 472 (ill.)

Mind and physical activity, *1:* 53–55, 57

Minerals in diet. *See* Vitamins and minerals

MMR (Measles-Mumps-Rubella), *2:* 238

Modeling, *3:* 448 (ill.), 448–449, 463–464

Model of the mouth of a tobacco user, *3:* 557 (ill.)

Monosodium glutamate (MSG), *2:* 229, 230

Mood disorders, *3:* 503–508, 504 (ill.), 507 (ill.)

Morissette, Alanis, *3:* 570

Morning after pill, *1:* 171

Morrison, Jim, *3:* 537

Morton, Richard, *3:* 564

Mosquito bites, *2:* 248, 260

Mowrer, O. H., *3:* 502

Mowrer, W. M., *3:* 502

MRI (Magnetic resonance imaging), *2:* 355, 356, 357 (ill.)

MSG (Monosodium glutamate), *2:* 229, 230

Munchausen, Baron Von, *3:* 522

Munchausen-by-proxy syndrome, *3:* 522

Munchausen syndrome, *3:* 522

Murphy, Brittany, *3:* 537

Muscles, *1:* 49–51

Music therapy, *3:* 471

Musical instruments, *3:* 427 (ill.)

Mydland, Brent, *3:* 537

MyPlate, *1:* 12–22, 13 (ill.)

National Organization For Women (NOW), *1:* 173 (ill.)

National Press Club (Washington, DC), *2:* 327 (ill.)

National Youth Violence Prevention Week, *3:* 425

Native American women and homeopathy, *2:* 369

Native Americans
   medical marijuana, *3:* 542
   naturopathy, *2:* 376, 377 (ill.)

Natural family planning, *1:* 167 (ill.)

Nature *vs.* nurture, *3:* 436–440

Naturopathy, *2:* 332, 376–381, 377 (ill.)

NBCC (National Board for Certified Counselors), *2:* 344

NCCAM (National Center for Complementary and Alternative Medicine), *2:* 303

Needle sharing, *3:* 540

Neighborhoods, *1:* 124–125, 125 (ill.)

Neurology, *2:* 350

The New Teenage Body Book (Tanner), *1:* 151–153, 152 (ill.), 155 (ill.), 156

Next Choice, *1:* 171

Next Choice One Dose, *1:* 171

Nicotine and nicotine-replacement products, *2:* 292–293, 293 (ill.), *3:* 553 (ill.), 553–554, 557 (ill.). *See also* Tobacco use

NIDA (National Institute on Drug Abuse), *2:* 274, 275, 276

Nietzsche, Friedrich, *3:* 459

NIMH (National Institute of Mental Health), *3:* 566

9/11 terrorist attacks, *3:* 520 (ill.)

Nitrogen dioxide (NO_2), *2:* 198, 203–204

Nocturnal emissions, *1:* 151

Nail care, *1:* 101–103

Narcissistic personality disorder, *3:* 526

Narcotics, *3:* 539–540

Nasal decongestants, *2:* 290, 298–299

National 9/11 Memorial, *3:* 520 (ill.)

National Association for Self-Esteem, *3:* 415, 416

National Board for Certified Counselors (NBCC), *2:* 344

National Center for Complementary and Alternative Medicine (NCCAM), *2:* 303

National Institute of Mental Health (NIMH), *3:* 566

National Institute on Drug Abuse (NIDA), *2:* 274, 275, 276

Nogier, Paul, *2:* 388

Non-H_2-Antagonists, *2:* 280

Non-ionizing radiation, *2:* 189

Nonconformity, *3:* 451

NRC (Nuclear Regulatory Committee), *2:* 191, 192

Nuclear medicine technologists, *2:* 358

Nuclear Regulatory Committee (NRC), *2:* 191, 192

Nurses
   advanced practice, *2:* 269, 359 (ill.), 359–361, *3:* 458 (ill.)
   certified nurse-midwives, 2, 360
   registered, *2:* 358–361, 359 (ill.)

N

Nurture *vs.* nature, *3:* 436–440
Nutrition, *1:* **1–42.** *See also* Vitamins and minerals
    breakfast, *1:* 41
    Dietary Guidelines for Americans, *1:* 6
    food allergies and intolerance, *1:* 37–40, 38 (ill.)
    food groups, *1:* 11
    healthful eating habits, *1:* 5, 5 (ill.), 22, 40–41
    independent eaters, *1:* 34 (ill.), 34–35
    junk food, *1:* 22–23
    MyPlate, *1:* 12–22, 13 (ill.)
    nutrients, *1:* 5–9
    snacking, *1:* 24–27, 25 (ill.), 26 (ill.)
    vegetarian and vegan diets, *1:* 35–37
    weight and body shape, *1:* 27–31, 28 (ill.),
      30 (ill.)
    weight management and dieting, *1:* 31–34
Nuts, *1:* 25 (ill.)

O

Obama, Barack, *2:* 313, 317 (ill.), *3:* 549
Obama, Michelle, *1:* 13 (ill.)
Obesity and overweight, *1:* 6, 11, 28 (ill.), 28–29
Observational learning, *3:* 447–449, 448 (ill.)
Obsessive-compulsive disorder (OCD), *3:* 516–518,
    517 (ill.), 574
Obstetrics, *2:* 350
Occupational Safety and Health Administration
    (OSHA), *2:* 192
Occupational therapists, *2:* 344–345
OCD (Obsessive-compulsive disorder), *3:* 516–518,
    517 (ill.), 574
ODD (Oppositional defiant disorder), *3:* 493–494
Oils, *1:* 20
Oliver, Jamie, *1:* 141
Olsen, Mary Kate, *3:* 570
Oncology, *2:* 350
Onychomycosis, *1:* 102
Operant conditioning, *3:* 446–447, 447 (ill.),
    462–463, 463 (ill.)
Operation Oak Tree, *3:* 472 (ill.)
Ophthalmology, *2:* 350
Oppositional defiant disorder (ODD), *3:* 493–494
Optometrists, *2:* 269, 345–346, 346 (ill.)

Oral and dental care, *1:* 95–98, 96 (ill.), 98 (ill.),
    2: 236, 337 (ill.)
Oral contraceptives, *1:* 167 (ill.), 168–169,
    169 (ill.)
Oral sex, *1:* 166
Organization, *3:* 443
Orthodontists, *2:* 337 (ill.)
Orthopedics, *2:* 350
OSHA (Occupational Safety and Health
    Administration), *2:* 192
Osler, William, *2:* 385
Osteoporosis, *1:* 19, 51–52
Otolaryngology, *2:* 350
Outdoor air pollution, *2:* 195–199, 196 (ill.),
    198 (ill.)
Outdoor injuries, *2:* 246–249
Over-the-counter drugs, *2:* 277, 278–279, 303–305,
    305 (ill.), 308 (ill.), *3:* 539
    common types, *2:* 279–291, 283 (ill.), 285 (ill.),
      288 (ill.)
    controversial or potentially dangerous, *2:* 292–301
    labels, *2:* 295–296
Overdoses and missed doses of medications,
    2: 272–274
Overheating, *1:* 72
Overweight and obesity, *1:* 6, 28 (ill.), 28–29
Ovulation, *1:* 154
OxyContin (oxycodone), *2:* 275
Ozone layer, *2:* 199

P

Pads, sanitary, *1:* 105–106, 107 (ill.)
Pain management, *2:* 282–284, 283 (ill.),
    3: 465–466
Palmer, B. J., *2:* 389
Palmer, Daniel David, *2:* 389
Paltrow, Gwyneth, *3:* 505
Panic attacks and panic disorder, *3:* 515–516
Paquin, Anna, *1:* 52
Paranoid personality disorder, *3:* 525
Parmertor, Danny, *3:* 421 (ill.)
Paronychia, *1:* 102
Particles and air pollution, *2:* 204

PAs (Physician assistants), *2:* 269, 359–361

Pasteur, Louis, *1:* 83

Patient advocates, *2:* 342

Patient Protection and Affordable Care Act (ACA), *2:* 313, 316, 317, 317 (ill.)

Pavlov, Ivan, *3:* 446

PCP (Phencyclidine), *3:* 546

PDD-NOS (Pervasive developmental disorder not otherwise specified), *3:* 498

Pediatrics, *2:* 350

Pedicures and manicures, *1:* 101

Peer pressure, *1:* 164–165, *3:* 414, 451

Pelvic inflammatory disease (PID), *1:* 176

Penises, *1:* 108–110, 109 (ill.), 150–151, 152, 152 (ill.)

Perfumes, colognes, and scented soaps and lotions, *1:* 83

Perls, Frederich S., *3:* 460–461

Perry, Matthew, *3:* 537

Person-centered therapy, *3:* 459–460

Personal care and hygiene, *1:* 77–112
  body basics, *1:* 80–83
  clothing, *1:* 110–111
  ears, *1:* 98–101
  genital care for females, *1:* 103–107, 107 (ill.)
  genital care for males, *1:* 108–110, 109 (ill.)
  hair, *1:* 88–95, 92 (ill.)
  health and, *2:* 236
  history of hygiene, *1:* 83
  nails, *1:* 101–103, 102 (ill.)
  sheets, towels, and washcloths, *1:* 111
  shoes, *1:* 111
  skin, *1:* 84–88
  teeth, *1:* 95–98, 96 (ill.), 98 (ill.), *2:* 236 (ill.)

Personal growth and development, *1:* 113–142
  developmental disorders, *1:* 139–141
  emotional intelligence, *1:* 138–139
  environment, *1:* 122–27, 123 (ill.), 124 (ill.), 125 (ill.), 126 (ill.)
  genetics, *1:* 116–122, 117 (ill.)
  intellectual development, *1:* 135–138
  physical development, *1:* 132–135, 133 (ill.), 134 (ill.)
  stages in personality development, *1:* 130 (ill.), 130–132, 132 (ill.)
  temperament and personality, *1:* 127–130

Personal unconscious, *3:* 456

Personality, *3:* 438–440, 440, 456

Personality development, *1:* 127, 130–132

Personality disorders, *3:* 524–526, 525 (ill.)

Persons with disabilities, *1:* 66 (ill.), *3:* 411, 414

Persons with eating disorders, *3:* 571 (ill.), 575 (ill.)

Pervasive developmental disorder not otherwise specified (PDD-NOS), *3:* 498

Pesticides, *2:* 192–195, 194 (ill.), 208–209, 212

Pets and self-esteem, *3:* 429–430

Petting (touching), *1:* 161

Peyote, *3:* 548

Pharmacists, *2:* 269, 271 (ill.), 347–348, 347 (ill.)

Pharmacotherapy, *3:* 466–467

Phelps, Michael, *1:* 141, *3:* 495

Phencyclidine (PCP), *3:* 546

Phobias, *3:* 513–515, 514 (ill.)

Phoenix, River, *3:* 537

Physical development, *1:* 132

Physical examinations and check-ups, *2:* 236–239

Physical fitness and exercise, *1:* 43–75. *See also* Sports
    activities that promote fitness, *1:* 55–66, 56 (ill.), 59 (ill.), 61 (ill.), 63 (ill.), 64 (ill.), 66 (ill.), 67 (ill.)
    in ancient times, *1:* 50
    benefits of, *1:* 46–55, 47 (ill.), 49 (ill.), 51 (ill.), 53 (ill.)
    exercising safely, *1:* 58, 60, 68–75, *2:* 233, 249–261
    health and, *2:* 231–232, 232 (ill.)
    physical activities as a permanent lifestyle, *1:* 67–75, 69 (ill.), 71 (ill.), 74 (ill.)
    types of, *1:* 49, 49 (ill.)

Physical medicine (naturopathy), *2:* 380

Physical therapists, *2:* 348–349, 349 (ill.)

Physician assistants (PAs), *2:* 269, 359–361

Physicians, *2:* 269, 320, 321 (ill.), 349–352, 351 (ill.)

PID (Pelvic inflammatory disease), *1:* 176

Piercings, *1:* 99, 99 (ill.)

Pill, The, *1:* 168–169, 167 (ill.), 169 (ill.)

Plan B, *1:* 171

Play age or preschool, *1:* 131

Playing, *1:* 47 (ill.), 61

PMS (Premenstrual syndrome), *1:* 158–159, *2:* 284, 292, 395

Point of service (POS) plan, *2:* 322
Poison oak and ivy, *2:* 247–248
Poisoning, *2:* 243–245
Polizzi, Nicole (Snooki), *3:* 570
Pollution
    indoor air, *2:* 199–212, 201 (ill.), 204 (ill.),
       206 (ill.)
    outdoor air, *2:* 195–199, 196 (ill.), 198 (ill.)
    water, *2:* 214 (ill.)
POS (Point of service) plan, *2:* 322
Pose2, *3:* 553 (ill.)
Post-traumatic stress disorder (PTSD), *3:* 518–521,
    520 (ill.)
Potassium in diet, *2:* 254
Prebiotics, *2:* 255
Preferred provider organization (PPO), *2:* 321
Pregnancy
    birth control, *1:* 167 (ill.), 167–171, 169 (ill.),
       170 (ill.)
    conception, *1:* 118
    endocrine disrupters, *2:* 213–214
    fetal development, *1:* 118–119
    lead-related problems, *2:* 208
    ovulation, *1:* 154
Premenstrual syndrome (PMS), *1:* 158–159, *2:* 284,
    292, 395
Preschool or play age, *1:* 131
Prescription drug abuse, *2:* 274–278, 277 (ill.)
Prescription drug safety, *2:* 272–273, 273 (ill.)
Prescription drugs, *2:* 267–274, 271 (ill.), 273 (ill.),
    296–297, 308 (ill.), 329–330, *3:* 539
Preteens and exercise, *1:* 59
Preventive care and first aid, *2:* 219–262
    dietary supplements, *2:* 251–255
    first aid, *2:* 256–261, 257 (ill.), 258 (ill.),
       259 (ill.), 291
    illness prevention, *2:* 224–239, 226 (ill.), 229 (ill.),
       232 (ill.), 235 (ill.), 236 (ill.), 238 (ill.)
    injury prevention, *2:* 239–251, 242 (ill.),
       244 (ill.), 247 (ill.)
    preventive medicine, *2:* 251–256
    responsibility for prevention, *2:* 221–223
Preventive medicine, *2:* 251–256
Pro-Ana and Pro-Mia web sites, *3:* 577
Probiotics, *2:* 255

Processed food, *2:* 226
Prostate gland, *1:* 150
Protein, *1:* 8
Protein group, *1:* 18–19
Psychedelic drugs, *3:* 547–550
Psychiatry, *2:* 350, 354
Psychoanalysis, *3:* 453 (ill.), 453–455
Psychodrama, *3:* 471–472, 472 (ill.)
Psychodynamic therapy, *3:* 455
Psychological medicine (naturopathy), *2:* 380
Psychologists, *2:* 269, 352–355
Psychology
    Adlerian, *3:* 457, 459
    analytical, *3:* 455–456
Psychotherapy, *3:* 452, 452 (ill.)
Psychotic disorders, *3:* 508–511, 510 (ill.)
PTSD (Post-traumatic stress disorder), *3:* 518–521,
    520 (ill.)
Puberty
    acne, *1:* 85–86, 86 (ill.), 87 (ill.), *2:* 286
    age of onset, *1:* 133, 134
    boys, *1:* 149–153, 152 (ill.)
    girls, *1:* 153–159, 155 (ill.), 157 (ill.)
Pubic lice, *1:* 180
Pulmonary physicians, *2:* 350
Purple cone-flowers (echinacea), *2:* 303 (ill.)
Pyromaniacs, *3:* 562

Q

Qi (life energy), *2:* 386
QMB (Qualified Medicare Beneficiaries Program),
    2: 323
Quaaludes, *3:* 541
Quaid, Dennis, *3:* 570
Qualified Medicare Beneficiaries Program (QMB),
    2: 323

R

Radiation, *2:* 189–192, 190 (ill.)
Radiographer, *2:* 356
Radiological technologists, *2:* 355–358, 357 (ill.)

Radiology, *2:* 350

Radner, Gilda, *3:* 570

Radon, *2:* 190, 192, 201–202, 204, 204 (ill.)

Ramone, Dee Dee, *3:* 537

Rape, date, *1:* 182

Rape crisis center, *1:* 181 (ill.)

Raspe, Rudolph Erich, *3:* 522

Rational-emotive behavior therapy, *3:* 462, 464–465

Raves, *3:* 545

Reading disorders, *3:* 495

Reality therapy, *3:* 466

Reflexology, *2:* 392, 394–397, 395 (ill.), 396 (ill.)

Registered nurses, *2:* 358–361, 359 (ill.)

Reich, Wilhelm, *3:* 469

Reid, Tara, *3:* 570

Renfro, Brad, *3:* 537

Respiratory problems, *2:* 202

Rett syndrome, *3:* 498

Reyes-Chian, Valeria, *1:* 66 (ill.)

Reye's syndrome, *2:* 298

Richie, Nicole, *1:* 52, *3:* 570

Rigby, Cathy, *3:* 570

Ringworm, nail, *1:* 102–103

Ritalin (methylphenidate), *2:* 276

Rivers, Joan, *3:* 570

Roberts, Eric, *3:* 503

Roe v. Wade (1973), *1:* 173, 174

Rogers, Carl, *3:* 459–460

Rohypnol, *1:* 182

Role models, *3:* 449

Roofies, *1:* 182

Rossi, Portia de, *3:* 570

Rotavirus (RV) vaccines, *2:* 238

Ruffies, *1:* 182

Running, *1:* 62

Russell, Gerald, *3:* 564

RV (Rotavirus) vaccines, *2:* 238

Ryder, Winona, *3:* 505

Sacks, Oliver, *3:* 499, 500

Salicylates, *2:* 231

Salk, Jonas, *2:* 374

Same-sex parents, *3:* 410

Sanitary pads, *1:* 105–106, 107 (ill.)

Sartre, Jean-Paul, *3:* 459

Savants, *3:* 500

Scalp conditions, *1:* 92–93

Scented soaps and lotions, *1:* 83

Schizophrenia, *3:* 508–511, 510 (ill.)

Schizotypal personality disorder, *3:* 525

School age children, *1:* 131, 133 (ill.), 133–134, 136–37, *2:* 233

School lunches, *1:* 34 (ill.)

School vending machines, *1:* 23, 23 (ill.)

School violence, *3:* 425

Seat belts, *2:* 224 (ill.)

Secondhand smoke, *2:* 200–202, 210, 210 (ill.), 228

Seizures, *2:* 261

Selenium in diet, *2:* 254–255

Self-concept, *3:* 406–412, 408 (ill.), 410 (ill.)

Self-confidence and self-esteem, *1:* 55

Self-esteem, *3:* 403–431

    building, *3:* 425–430, 427 (ill.)

    cyberbullying, *3:* 424 (ill.)

    family, *3:* 409–412, 410 (ill.)

    friends, *3:* 417–420, 418 (ill.)

    harmful actions and behaviors, *3:* 420–421

    healthy self-esteem, *3:* 415–416, 416 (ill.)

    low self-esteem, *3:* 412–415, 413 (ill.)

    self-concept, *3:* 405–412, 408 (ill.)

    unhealthy high self-esteem, *3:* 417

    violent behavior, *3:* 421 (ill.), 421–425, 423 (ill.)

Self-harm, *3:* 561 (ill.), 561–562

Self-injury, *3:* 561 (ill.), 561–562

Separation and divorce, *3:* 411

Separation anxiety, *3:* 512

Set point theory of weight, *1:* 28–29

Sex addiction, *3:* 563

Sex therapy, *3:* 474

Sexual harassment and abuse, *1:* 180–183, 181 (ill.)

Sexual intercourse, *1:* 164–166

Sexuality, *1:* 143–183

    birth control, *1:* 167 (ill.), 167–171, 169 (ill.), 170 (ill.)

    eating disorders, *3:* 576–577

kissing, dating and physical attraction, *1:* 159–164, 161 (ill.), 162 (ill.)

pregnancy, *1:* 171–175, 173 (ill.), 175 (ill.)

puberty, *1:* 149

puberty in boys, *1:* 149–153, 152 (ill.)

puberty in girls, *1:* 153–159, 155 (ill.), 157 (ill.)

sex, *1:* 164–166

sexual harassment and abuse, *1:* 180–183, 181 (ill.)

sexually transmitted diseases (STDs), *1:* 168, 169, 170, 175–180, 178 (ill.)

talking about sex, *1:* 146–149, 148 (ill.)

Sexually transmitted diseases (STDs), *1:* 168, 169, 170, 175–180, 178 (ill.)

Shampoo and conditioner, *1:* 91–92

Shaving, *1:* 93, 93 (ill.)

Sheedy, Ally, *3:* 570

Sheldon, William H., *1:* 27

Shiatsu, *2:* 393

Shields, Brooke, *3:* 505

Shoe care, *1:* 111

Sierra Club, *2:* 187

Simpson, Ashlee, *3:* 570

Skiing and snowboarding, *1:* 62, 67 (ill.)

Skin cancer, *2:* 237

Skin care, *1:* 84–88, 86 (ill.), 87 (ill.)

Skinner, B. F., *3:* 447, 462, 463 (ill.)

Sleep aids, *2:* 294, 301, *3:* 540–541

Sleep and health, *1:* 55, *2:* 234–236, 235 (ill.)

Sleep and mental health, *3:* 480

SLMB (Specified Low Income Medicare Beneficiary), *2:* 323

Slovak, Hillel, *3:* 537

"Smiles" (designer drug), *3:* 549

Smith, Anna Nicole, *3:* 537

Smith, Harriet, *3:* 571 (ill.)

Smith, Will, *1:* 141

Smoked food, *2:* 226

Smoking, *See* Tobacco use

Snacking, *1:* 24–27, 25 (ill.)

Snakebites, *2:* 248

Snowboarding and skiing, *1:* 62, 67 (ill.)

Soaps and lotions, *1:* 83

Soccer, *1:* 56 (ill.)

Social anxiety disorder, *3:* 512–513

Social workers, *2:* 269, 361–362

Soda, sports drinks, and other sugar-sweetened beverages, *1:* 11

Softball, *1:* 51 (ill.), 69

Somatoform disorders, *3:* 521–522

Sonographers, *2:* 356–357

Specified Low Income Medicare Beneficiary (SLMB), *2:* 323

Speech language pathologists, *2:* 362–363

Sperm, journey of the, *1:* 150

SPF (sun protection factor), *1:* 87–88

Spice (designer drug), *3:* 549–550

Spider bites, *2:* 248, 249, 260

Spiders, fear of, *3:* 514 (ill.)

Sports. *See also* **Physical fitness and exercise**

baseball, *1:* 69

biking, *1:* 57–58

boot camp, *1:* 63

boxing, *1:* 63–64

dance, *1:* 56–57, 58, 59 (ill.), *3:* 471

extreme, *1:* 67

football, *1:* 71 (ill.)

gymnastics, *1:* 53 (ill.), 58–59

head injuries, *1:* 70–72, 71 (ill.)

helmets, *2:* 249

hiking, *1:* 59–60

ice skating, *1:* 60

in-line skating, *1:* 60, 69 (ill.)

injuries, *1:* 72–74, *2:* 249–251, 250 (ill.)

martial arts, *1:* 60–61

the mind and, *1:* 57

and safety, *1:* 58, 60, 68–75, *2:* 233, 249–261

skiing, *1:* 62

snowboarding, *1:* 62, 67 (ill.)

softball, *1:* 69

special equipment, *1:* 69

swimming, *1:* 62–63, 63 (ill.), 100

team, *1:* 65

tennis, *1:* 65, 66 (ill.)

Title IX, *1:* 64

walking, *1:* 65–66

yoga, *1:* 66–67, 74 (ill.), 159, *2:* 398–401, 400 (ill.), *3:* 467 (ill.), 467–468

Sports drinks, *1:* 11

Sports massage, *2:* 392

Sports nutrition supplements, *2:* 302

Sprains and strains, *2:* 260

St. John's wort (hypericum perforatum), *2:* 308

Stanford-Binet Intelligence Scale, *3:* 449–450

Starr, Ellen, *2:* 362

Starr, Mike, *3:* 537

STDs (Sexually transmitted diseases), *1:* 168, 169, 170, 175–180, 178 (ill.)

Stern, Lynn, *3:* 443

Stewart, Kristen, *1:* 52

Stimulants (drugs), *3:* 543–546, 545 (ill.)

Stimulation of children, *3:* 445–446

Stings and bites, *2:* 248–249, 260

Stone, Emma, *1:* 52

Stoves, heaters, fireplaces, and chimneys, *2:* 202, 210–211

Strains and sprains, *2:* 260

Strength, *1:* 49–51

Stress management, *1:* 55, *2:* 232–234, *3:* 443, 465

Stuckman, Duane, *3:* 472 (ill.)

Study habits, *3:* 439 (ill.)

Stuttering, *3:* 502–503

Substance abuse, *2:* 274–278, 277 (ill.), 333–334, *3:* 535–539, 537 (ill.), 576

Substance abuse counselors, *2:* 344

Sugar, *1:* 24, *3:* 555

Sugar-sweetened beverages, *1:* 11

Sugaring, *1:* 94

Suicide, *2:* 241, 242, *3:* 506

Sulfites, *2:* 230–231

Sulfur dioxide (SO$_2$), *2:* 197, 198

Sun protection, *1:* 87–88, 89 (ill.)

Sun protection factor (SPF), *1:* 87–88

Superego, *3:* 454

Support groups, *3:* 479

Supreme Court, *1:* 173, 174, 175 (ill.)

Swimmer's ear, *1:* 100

Swimming, *1:* 62–63, 63 (ill.)

Syphilis, *1:* 178

Szasz, Thomas, *3:* 420

T

Takeout food, *1:* 26 (ill.)

Tamper-evident packaging (TEP), *2:* 304–305

Tampons, *1:* 105–106, 107 (ill.)

Tanner, J. M., *1:* 151, 151–153, 152 (ill.), 155 (ill.), 156

Taoism, *2:* 386

Tar accumulated in the lungs by a smoker, *3:* 557 (ill.)

TB (Tuberculosis), *2:* 239

TCM (Traditional Chinese medicine), *2:* 380, 381–385, 382 (ill.), 383 (ill.)

Tdap (Tetanus-Diphtheria-Pertussis) vaccine, *2:* 238

Team sport, *1:* 65

Teeth, *1:* 95–97

Temperament and personality, 127

Telemedicine, *2:* 329, 329 (ill.)

Tennis, *1:* 65, 66 (ill.)

TEP (Tamper-evident packaging), *2:* 304–305

Terman, Lewis, *3:* 449

Testosterone, *1:* 149

Tetanus-Diphtheria-Pertussis (Tdap), *2:* 238

Therapeutic asanas, *2:* 399

Therapists, choosing a, *3:* 459

Thinspiration, *3:* 577

Thirdhand smoke, *2:* 201, 210, 210 (ill.)

Thomson, Samuel, *2:* 371

Thorndike, E. L., *3:* 462

Thornton, Billy Bob, *3:* 570

Ticks, *2:* 248

Timberlake, Justin, *3:* 495

Tisdale, Ashley, *1:* 52

Title IX, *1:* 64, 64 (ill.)

TIV (influenza vaccines), *2:* 238

Tobacco use. *See also* Nicotine and nicotine-replacement products

    environmental/secondhand tobacco smoke, *2:* 200–202, 210, 210 (ill.), 227

    illness prevention and, *2:* 227–228

    self-esteem and, *3:* 413 (ill.)

    thirdhand smoke, *2:* 201, 210, 210 (ill.)

Toddlers, *1:* 131, 132–133, 136, *3:* 441

Toenails

    ingrown, *1:* 101

    ringworm, *1:* 102–103

Tooth care, *1:* 95–98, 96 (ill.), 98 (ill.)

Topical medications, *2:* 285 (ill.), 285–286

Tourette syndrome, *3:* 501

Toynbee Hall (London, England), *2:* 362

Traditional Chinese medicine, *2:* 380, 381–385, 382 (ill.), 383 (ill.)

Transference, *3:* 454–455

Trichomoniasis, *1:* 104
Tripping, *3:* 547
True Life (MTV), *3:* 510 (ill.)
Tuberculosis (TB), *2:* 239
Turner, Ike, *3:* 537
Tweezing, *1:* 93–94
Twins, *1:* 119, *3:* 439, 509
Twitter, *3:* 425
Tyler, Liv, *1:* 141

U

Unconscious, collective, *3:* 455, 456
Unemployment, *3:* 411
University of Connecticut Migrant Farm Worker
    Clinics, *2:* 351 (ill.)
University of Rhode Island (South Kingstown, RI),
    2: 347 (ill.)
Unplanned pregnancy, *1:* 171–175
Urethra, *1:* 153
Urinary tract infections (UTIs), *1:* 104
Urology, *2:* 350
U.S. Centers for Disease Control and Prevention. *See*
    Centers for Disease Control and Prevention (CDC)
U.S. Congress, *2:* 187, 275, *3:* 549
U.S. Department of Agriculture (USDA), *1:* 6, 11, 16
U.S. Department of Defense (DOD), *2:* 192
U.S. Department of Education, *3:* 425
U.S. Department of Energy (DOE), *2:* 192
U.S. Department of Health and Human Services
    (HHS), *1:* 11, *2:* 192, 215, 275
U.S. Department of Transportation (DOT), *2:* 192
U.S. Drug Enforcement Administration (DEA), *3:* 549
U.S. Environmental Protection Agency (EPA). *See*
    Environmental Protection Agency (EPA)
U.S. Food and Drug Administration. *See* Food and
    Drug Administration (FDA)
U.S. Health Resources and Services Administration,
    3: 425
U.S. Preventive Service Task Force, *2:* 252–253
U.S. Supreme Court, *1:* 173, 174, 175 (ill.)
USA Ski Team's Mobile Nutrition Center, *2:* 226 (ill.)
Usher, *1:* 52
Uterus, *1:* 154
UTIs (urinary tract infections), *1:* 104

V

VA hospital (Prescott, AZ), *2:* 377 (ill.)
Vaccinations, *2:* 236, 238, 238 (ill.), 239
Vagina, *1:* 153–154
Vaginal infections, *1:* 103–104
Vaginal rings, *1:* 167 (ill.)
Varicella (VAR), *2:* 238
Vegan and vegetarian diets, *1:* 19, 35–37
Vegetable group. *See* Fruits and vegetables
Vegetarian and vegan diets, *1:* 19, 35–37
Vending machines in schools, *1:* 23, 23 (ill.)
Veterans and PTSD, *3:* 519
Veterans' hospital (Prescott, AZ), *2:* 377 (ill.)
VetoViolence, *3:* 425
Vicodin, *2:* 274–275
Video games, *3:* 559 (ill.)
Viera, Meredith, *3:* 570
Violent behavior, *2:* 241–243, *3:* 421 (ill.),
    421–425, 423 (ill.)
Vision and hearing tests, *2:* 239
Visualization, *3:* 443
Vitamins and minerals. *See also* **Nutrition**
    dairy food, *1:* 17
    in diet, *1:* 37 (ill.), *2:* 225–226, 252–255
    dietary supplements, *2:* 301–303, 302 (ill.),
        306–308
    minerals, *1:* 9, *2:* 254–255
    vitamins, *1:* 8–9, *2:* 253
Volatile organic compounds (VOCs), *2:* 196–197
Volunteering, *3:* 429, 429 (ill.)
Vulva, *1:* 153

W

Wagner, Rachel, *1:* 66 (ill.)
Walk In Medical Clinic (Venice Beach, CA), *3:* 542 (ill.)
Walking, *1:* 65–66
Warts, *1:* 179
Water in diet, *1:* 9, 10, 10 (ill.), *2:* 228, 229 (ill.)
Water safety, *2:* 246–247, 247 (ill.)
Watson, James, *1:* 120
Waxing, *1:* 94
Weight-bearing exercise, *1:* 51, 51 (ill.), 74 (ill.)

Weight loss aids, *1:* 32–34, *2:* 294–295, 301
Weight management and dieting, *1:* 31–34
Welsh, Mikey, *3:* 537
Wesley Community Center (Phoenix, AZ), *2:* 316 (ill.)
Willis, Bruce, *3:* 503
Wilson, Nancy, *3:* 503
Wilson, Owen, *3:* 505
Winehouse, Amy, *3:* 537, 537 (ill.)
Winfrey, Oprah, *3:* 570
Winslet, Kate, *3:* 570
Withdrawal from drugs, *3:* 540
Woody, Allen, *3:* 537
World Wildlife Fund (WWF), *2:* 187
Writing and memory, *3:* 443

X

X rays, *2:* 390 (ill.)

Y

Yang and yin, *2:* 386
Yeast infection medicine, *2:* 287
Yeast infections, *1:* 104
Yin and yang, *2:* 386
Yoga
    alternative medicine, *2:* 398–401, 400 (ill.)
    asthma, *2:* 401
    as exercise, *1:* 52, 66–67, 74 (ill.), 159
    mental health, *3:* 467 (ill.), 467–468
Yungborn Nature Cure Health Resort (New York),
    2: 379

Z

Zeta-Jones, Catherine, *3:* 505
Zinc in diet, *2:* 255